Hand Infections

Editors

JOHN R. FOWLER
RICK TOSTI

HAND CLINICS

www.hand.theclinics.com

Consulting Editor
KEVIN C. CHUNG

August 2020 • Volume 36 • Number 3

ELSEVIER

1600 John F. Kennedy Boulevard • Suite 1800 • Philadelphia, Pennsylvania, 19103-2899

http://www.theclinics.com

HAND CLINICS Volume 36, Number 3
August 2020 ISSN 0749-0712, ISBN-13: 978-0-323-71348-1

Editor: Lauren Boyle
Developmental Editor: Kristen Helm

Hand Clinics (ISSN 0749-0712) is published quarterly by Elsevier Inc., 360 Park Avenue South, New York, NY 10010-1710. Months of publication are February, May, August, and November. Business and Editorial Offices: 1600 John F. Kennedy Blvd., Ste. 1800, Philadelphia, PA 19103-2899. Customer Service Office: 3251 Riverport Lane, Maryland Heights, MO 63043. Periodicals postage paid at New York, NY and at additional mailing offices. Subscription price is $439.00 per year (domestic individuals), $854.00 per year (domestic institutions), $100.00 per year (domestic students/residents), $501.00 per year (Canadian individuals), $994.00 per year (Canadian institutions), $562.00 per year (international individuals), $994.00 per year (international institutions), $256.00 (international students/residents), and $100.00 (Canadian students/residents). Foreign air speed delivery is included in all *Clinics* subscription prices. All prices are subject to change without notice. **POSTMASTER:** Send address changes to *Hand Clinics*, Elsevier Health Sciences Division, Subscription Customer Service, 3251 Riverport Lane, Maryland Heights, MO 63043. Customer Service (orders, claims, online, change of address): Elsevier Health Sciences Division, Subscription **Customer Service, 3251 Riverport Lane, Maryland Heights, MO 63043. Tel: 1-800-654-2452 (U.S. and Canada); 314-447-8871 (outside U.S. and Canada). Fax: 314-447-8029. E-mail: journalscustomerservice-usa@elsevier.com (for print support); journalsonlinesupport-usa@elsevier.com (for online support).**

Reprints. For copies of 100 or more of articles in this publication, please contact the Commercial Reprints Department, Elsevier Inc., 360 Park Avenue South, New York, New York 10010-1710. Tel.: 212-633-3874; Fax: 212-633-3820; E-mail: reprints@elsevier.com.

Hand Clinics is covered in *MEDLINE/PubMed (Index Medicus), Current Contents/Clinical Medicine, EMBASE/Excerpta Medica,* and *ISI/BIOMED.*

Contributors

CONSULTING EDITOR

KEVIN C. CHUNG, MD, MS
Charles B. G. de Nancrede Professor of
Surgery, Professor of Plastic Surgery and
Orthopaedic Surgery, Chief of Hand Surgery,
Michigan Medicine, Assistant Dean for Faculty
Affairs, Associate Director of Global REACH,
University of Michigan Medical School, Ann
Arbor, Michigan

EDITORS

RICK TOSTI, MD
Hand, Wrist, Elbow, and Microvascular
Surgeon, Philadelphia Hand to Shoulder
Center, Assistant Professor of Orthopaedic
Surgery, Thomas Jefferson University,
Philadelphia, Pennsylvania

JOHN R. FOWLER, MD
Assistant Dean, University of Pittsburgh School
of Medicine, Associate Professor, Department
of Orthopedics, Associate Program Director,
Hand and Upper Extremity Surgery Fellowship,
Pittsburgh, Pennsylvania

AUTHORS

KAMAL ADDAGATLA, MD
Resident, Division of Plastic Surgery, Cooper
University Health Care, Camden,
New Jersey

ABDO BACHOURA, MD
Hand and Upper Extremity Fellow, Philadelphia
Hand to Shoulder Center, Thomas Jefferson
University Hospital, Philadelphia,
Pennsylvania

JAMES BARGER, MD
Resident, Division of Hand Surgery,
Department of Orthopaedic Surgery,
Massachusetts General Hospital, MGH
Orthopaedic Hand Surgery, Yawkey Center for
Outpatient Care, Boston, Massachusetts

NEAL CHEN, MD
Attending Surgeon, Division of Hand Surgery,
Department of Orthopaedic Surgery,
Massachusetts General Hospital, MGH
Orthopaedic Hand Surgery, Yawkey Center for
Outpatient Care, Boston, Massachusetts

BRIAN CHENOWETH, MD
Assistant Professor, University of Oklahoma,
Oklahoma City, Oklahoma

KEVIN C. CHUNG, MD, MS
Charles B. G. de Nancrede Professor of
Surgery, Professor of Plastic Surgery and
Orthopaedic Surgery, Chief of Hand
Surgery, Michigan Medicine, Assistant
Dean for Faculty Affairs, Associate Director
of Global REACH, University of
Michigan Medical School, Ann Arbor,
Michigan

ZACHARY J. FINLEY, MD
Department of Orthopaedic Surgery, Tulane
University School of Medicine, New Orleans,
Louisiana

MARY PATRICIA FOX, MD
Fellow, Department of Orthopaedic Surgery,
Philadelphia Hand to Shoulder Center, Thomas
Jefferson University, Philadelphia,
Pennsylvania

ROHIT GARG, MBBS
Attending Surgeon, Division of Hand Surgery,
Department of Orthopaedic Surgery,
Massachusetts General Hospital, MGH
Orthopaedic Hand Surgery, Yawkey Center for
Outpatient Care, Boston, Massachusetts

TETYANA GORBACHOVA, MD
Section Chief, Musculoskeletal Imaging,
Clinical Associate Professor, Department of
Radiology, Einstein Healthcare Network,
Jefferson Medical College, Philadelphia,
Pennsylvania

KANU GOYAL, MD
Department of Orthopaedic Surgery, Hand and
Upper Extremity Center, The Ohio State
Wexner Medical Center, Columbus, Ohio

BEN K. GUNDLACH, MD
Orthopaedic Surgery Resident, Department of
Orthopaedic Surgery, University of Michigan,
Ann Arbor, Michigan

JESSICA M. INTRAVIA, MD
Philadelphia Hand to Shoulder Center,
Philadelphia, Pennsylvania

SIDNEY M. JACOBY, MD
Assistant Professor, Department of
Orthopaedic Surgery, Philadelphia Hand to
Shoulder Center, Thomas Jefferson University,
Philadelphia, Pennsylvania

NICOLE J. JARRETT, MD, FACS
Assistant Professor of Surgery, Division of
Plastic Surgery, Cooper University Health
Care, Camden, New Jersey

SARA LOW, MD
Department of Orthopedic Surgery, Einstein
Healthcare Network, Philadelphia,
Pennsylvania

JOSHUA LUGINBUHL, MD
Resident, Department of Orthopaedics and
Sports Medicine, Temple University Hospital,
Philadelphia, Pennsylvania

GLEB MEDVEDEV, MD
Assistant Professor, Department of
Orthopaedic Surgery, Tulane University School
of Medicine, New Orleans, Louisiana

ATLEE MELILLO, MD
Resident, Division of Plastic Surgery, Cooper
University Health Care, Camden, New Jersey

MEREDITH N. OSTERMAN, MD
Philadelphia Hand to Shoulder Center,
Philadelphia, Pennsylvania

VANESSA PROKUSKI, MD
Hand Surgeon, Philadelphia Hand to Shoulder
Center, Thomas Jefferson University Hospital,
Philadelphia, Pennsylvania; Orthopedic
Surgeon, Orthopedic Care Physicians
Network, Raynham, Massachusetts

JAMES S. RAPHAEL, MD
Chairman, Department of Orthopedic Surgery,
Director, Hand and Upper Extremity Division,
Einstein Healthcare Network, Philadelphia,
Pennsylvania

MARK S. REKANT, MD
Associate Professor, Philadelphia Hand to
Shoulder Center, Associate Professor,
Department of Orthopaedic Surgery, Thomas
Jefferson University, Philadelphia,
Pennsylvania; Admin Asst, Patricia Lincke,
Cherry Hill, New Jersey

SARAH E. SASOR, MD
Assistant Professor, Department of Plastic
Surgery, Medical College of Wisconsin,
Milwaukee, Wisconsin

MARK K. SOLARZ, MD
Assistant Professor, Department of
Orthopaedics and Sports Medicine, Temple
University Hospital, Philadelphia, Pennsylvania

AMY L. SPEECKAERT, MD, MS
Department of Orthopaedic Surgery, Hand and
Upper Extremity Center, The Ohio State
Wexner Medical Center, Columbus, Ohio

ADAM STROHL, MD
Hand Surgeon, Departments of Orthopedics,
Plastic and Reconstructive Surgery,
Philadelphia Hand to Shoulder Center, Thomas
Jefferson University Hospital, Philadelphia,
Pennsylvania

JOSEPH F. STYRON, MD, PhD
Assistant Professor of Surgery, Cleveland
Clinic, Cleveland Clinic Lerner College of

Medicine of Case Western Reserve University, Cleveland, Ohio

RYAN TARR, DO
Philadelphia Hand to Shoulder Center, Philadelphia, Pennsylvania

RICK TOSTI, MD
Hand, Wrist, Elbow, and Microvascular Surgeon, Philadelphia Hand to Shoulder Center, Assistant Professor of Orthopaedic Surgery, Thomas Jefferson University, Philadelphia, Pennsylvania

FREDERICK WANG, MD
Fellow, Division of Hand Surgery, Department of Orthopaedic Surgery, Massachusetts General Hospital, MGH Orthopaedic Hand

Surgery, Yawkey Center for Outpatient Care, Boston, Massachusetts

COLIN M. WHITAKER, MD
Department of Orthopedic Surgery, Einstein Healthcare Network, Philadelphia, Pennsylvania

CHRIS WILLIAMSON, MD
Hand and Upper Extremity Division, Einstein Healthcare Network, Department of Orthopedic Surgery, East Norriton, Pennsylvania

DAVID S. ZELOUF, MD
Philadelphia Hand to Shoulder Center, Assistant Professor, Thomas Jefferson University Hospital, Philadelphia, Pennsylvania

Contents

> Upper extremity infections are common. Most infections can be effectively treated with minor surgical procedures and/or oral antibiotics; however, inappropriate or delayed care can result in significant, long-term morbidity. The basic principles of treating hand infections were described more than a century ago and most remain relevant today. Immunosuppressant medications, chronic health conditions such as diabetes and human immunodeficiency virus, and public health problems like intravenous drug use, have changed the landscape of hand infections and provide new challenges in treatment.

> Hand infections can lead to significant morbidity if not treated promptly. Most of these infections, such as abscesses, tenosynovitis, cellulitis, and necrotizing fasciitis, can be diagnosed clinically. Laboratory values, such as white blood cell count, erythrocyte sedimentation rate, C-reactive protein, and recently, procalcitonin and interleukin-6, are helpful in supporting the diagnosis and trending disease progression. Radiographs should be obtained in all cases of infection. Ultrasound is a dynamic study that can provide quick evaluation of deeper structures but is operator dependent. Computed tomographic and MRI studies are useful for evaluating deep space or bony infections and preoperative surgical planning.

> The rates of methicillin-resistant infections in the hand and upper extremity approach 50% in many facilities. In addition, multidrug resistance is beginning to include clindamycin. This article discusses the history, prevalence, and treatment of both community-acquired and health care–associated methicillin-resistant Staphylococcus aureus in regard to hand infections.

> A high index of suspicion coupled with excellent knowledge of hand anatomy and function allows for accurate diagnosis and effective management of deep space infections. This article describes surgical approaches for closed-space infections. Drainage, debridement, and intraoperative irrigation are initial steps along with the decision for continuous postoperative irrigation based on intraoperative findings. Focused and thorough postoperative evaluation and antibiotics lead to successful management of these soft tissue deep abscesses. An experienced hand therapist

should be involved early in recovery process to guide wound care along with passive assisted and active range of motion exercises of the wrist and digits.

James Barger, Rohit Garg, Frederick Wang, and Neal Chen

The fingertip is the most common site of infections in the hand, which frequently are encountered by surgeons, dermatologists, and emergency and primary providers. Their mismanagement may have serious consequences. This review discusses the unique anatomy of the volar fingertip pulp and perionychium and reviews pathophysiology and treatment of acute and chronic paronychia, including the decision for surgical versus medical management, choice of antibiotics, incisional techniques, and postincisional care. Felons and the evidence regarding their management are reviewed. Several infectious, rheumatologic, and oncologic conditions that may mimic common fingertip infections and about which the managing provider must be aware are presented.

Kanu Goyal and Amy L. Speeckaert

Pyogenic flexor tenosynovitis is a closed-space infection that can lead to a devastating loss of finger and hand function. It can spread rapidly into the palm, distal forearm, other digits, and nearby joints. Healthy individuals may present with no signs of systemic illness and often deny any penetrating trauma or inoculation. Early diagnosis and prompt treatment are required to preserve the digit and prevent morbidity and loss of hand function. Many treatment options have been described, although all share 2 common principles: evacuation of the infection and tailored postoperative antibiotic treatment with close monitoring to ensure clinical improvement.

Brian Chenoweth

Infections in the joints of the hand and wrist carry the risk of significant morbidity. Common presenting symptoms include joint redness, swelling, and pseudoparalysis that occurs several days following a penetrating trauma. Diagnostic workup should be expedited, including a laboratory evaluation and arthrocentesis. Imaging, including radiographs, ultrasound, computed tomography, and/or MRI, are helpful tools in diagnosis. Once infection is identified, prompt surgical debridement and antibiotics are required. Once the infection has been managed, hand therapy is initiated to decrease the risk of stiffness. Stiffness is the most common complication following infection; additional reported complications include arthritis, ankylosis, and amputation."

Atlee Melillo, Kamal Addagatla, and Nicole J. Jarrett

Necrotizing soft tissue infections of the upper extremity have varying microbiologies and etiologies. Risk factors for development include diabetes mellitus, intravenous drug use, peripheral arterial disease, smoking, alcohol abuse, and immunocompromised state. Although clinical examination is the mainstay of diagnosis, laboratory tests and imaging can aid in diagnosis. Surgical débridements usually are needed for treatment, with resultant defects that often require reconstruction. Rates of amputation are reported as 22% to 37.5% and mortality from necrotizing soft tissue infections of the upper extremity from 22% to 34%. Prompt surgical and antimicrobial treatment is necessary to decrease risk of loss of limb or life.

include healing by primary or secondary intention, skin grafts, local flaps, and distant flaps. Negative pressure wound therapy and acellular dermal matrices can also aid in coverage.

Infections are an important source of morbidity in pediatric hands that come from frequent exposure to mouths and other dangers while exploring the world. Although Staphylococcus aureus is still the most common organism in pediatric hand infections, it is less common than in adults because pediatric patients are more likely to develop mixed aerobic/anaerobic infections or group A Streptococcus pyogenes infection. Pediatric patients with open physes potentially may sustain Seymour fractures of the distal phalanges that may become infected and sources for osteomyelitis if not recognized early.

Mycobacterial hand infections are uncommon. These infections have an indolent course and are marked by variable and nonspecific presentations, often leading to diagnostic and treatment delays. The pathogens involved in mycobacterial hand infections include Mycobacterium tuberculosis complex, atypical mycobacteria, and M leprae. Initial treatment involves a combination of long-term antibiotics and surgical d_ebridement to cure the infection. Reconstructive procedures aid in restoring hand function lost secondary to the disease.

HAND CLINICS

SERIES OF RELATED INTEREST:

Clinics in Plastic Surgery
https://www.plasticsurgery.theclinics.com/

Orthopedic Clinics of North America
https://www.orthopedic.theclinics.com/

Physical Medicine and Rehabilitation Clinics of North America
https://www.pmr.theclinics.com/

THE CLINICS ARE AVAILABLE ONLINE!
Access your subscription at:
www.theclinics.com

HAND CLINICS

SERIES OF RELATED INTEREST

Preface

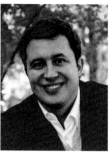
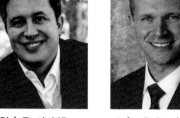

Rick Tosti, MD   John R. Fowler, MD

Editors

Prior to the discovery of the penicillin, infectious disease was a leading cause of death in the young and old and in both developed and underdeveloped countries. Since the Great Wars, medical science has evolved treatments that have greatly reduced the burden on humanity and have made it possible to cure many infections. However, as our treatments have evolved, so have microorganisms. Whereas once methicillin-resistant *Staphylococcus aureus* was confined to rare case reports, community-acquired infections with multidrug resistance have become the most commonly encountered pathogens in some regions and present a new challenge. Moreover, newer developments in treatments for autoimmune disease, transplant medicine, and human immunodeficiency virus have resulted in longer living immunocompromised individuals, who are known to be susceptible to a variety of atypical infections.

Despite the perception that treating infections has become routine, it is nevertheless necessary for the physician to recognize the present challenges and recommend a course of action. Although many innovations have greatly eased the burden of both the patient and the doctor, the threat of destruction to life and limb caused by infections remains. Fortunately, medical science has progressed to keep pace with the demands of a new era. Imaging and laboratory techniques have enhanced our ability to make a diagnosis. Advancements in antibiotic therapies have augmented the potential to eradicate severe infections. And finally, modern surgical debridement and wound management protocols may restore a functional limb. The collection of articles presented herein was designed as an overview for the current physician to navigate modern challenges with contemporary solutions.

Rick Tosti, MD
Philadelphia Hand to Shoulder Center
950 Pulaski Drive
King of Prussia, PA 19406, USA

John R. Fowler, MD
Department of Orthopedics
Hand and Upper Extremity Surgery Fellowship
University of Pittsburgh School of Medicine
Pittsburgh, PA, USA

E-mail addresses:
rjtosti@gmail.com (R. Tosti)
fowlerjr@upmc.edu (J.R. Fowler)

Hand Infections
Epidemiology and Public Health Burden

Ben K. Gundlach, MD[a],*, Sarah E. Sasor, MD[b], Kevin C. Chung, MD, MS[c]

KEYWORDS

- Hand infections • IVDU infections • Diabetic upper extremity infections • Infection epidemiology
- Infection public health

KEY POINTS

- Most hand infections are the result of direct trauma.
- Community-acquired methicillin-resistant *Staphylococcus aureus* is the most common organism isolated in upper extremity infections.
- Chronic health conditions, such as diabetes and human immunodeficiency virus, and medical immunosuppression predispose patients to common and atypical hand infections.

INTRODUCTION

Hand infections and their sequelae are a significant public health burden worldwide. Even when treated appropriately, infections can result in scarring, joint contractures, stiffness, and chronic pain. Although the field of hand surgery has evolved over the past century, infections of the hand, their causes, and treatments remain largely unchanged. Prompt diagnosis, surgical debridement, and antibiotic coverage remain the standard of care. As medical treatments for complex diseases improve, patients with chronic diseases are surviving longer. Identification of infection in immunosuppressed patients can be difficult because typical signs and symptoms are often lacking. Public health problems such as intravenous drug use lead to new challenges in treating patients with acute hand infections. The purpose of this article was to review the epidemiology and social impact of upper extremity infections.

HISTORY

Acute Phlegmons of the Hand, published in 1905 by Dr Allen Kanavel, was one of the first anatomic studies of the hand. Dr Kanavel (1874–1938) worked as a general surgeon in Chicago, IL, and cared for many patients with hand infections. Through repetition, he noticed predictable patterns. Using anatomic cross-sectioning and plaster-of-Paris injection studies, he defined the "5 great spaces" of the hand: dorsal subcutaneous, dorsal subaponeurotic, hypothenar, thenar, and middle palmar spaces.[1] Kanavel's work culminated with the publication of *Infections of the Hand*[2] in 1912, in which he systematically describes various infections and their management (**Fig. 1**).

EPIDEMIOLOGY

Data on the overall epidemiology of hand infections are scarce. Unique injury data, such as the

[a] Department of Orthopaedic Surgery, University of Michigan, 1500 East Medical Center Drive, 2912 Taubman Center, SPC 5328, Ann Arbor, MI 48109, USA; [b] Department of Plastic Surgery, Medical College of Wisconsin, Tosa Health Center, 2nd floor, 1155 N Mayfair Road, Wauwatosa, WI 53226, USA; [c] Department of Surgery, Section of Plastic Surgery, University of Michigan, Michigan Medicine, University of Michigan Medical School, 1500 East Medical Center Drive, 2130 Taubman Center, SPC 5340, Ann Arbor, MI 48109, USA
* Corresponding author.
E-mail address: bgundlac@med.umich.edu

Hand Clin 36 (2020) 275–283
https://doi.org/10.1016/j.hcl.2020.03.001

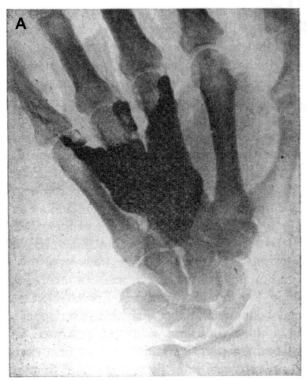
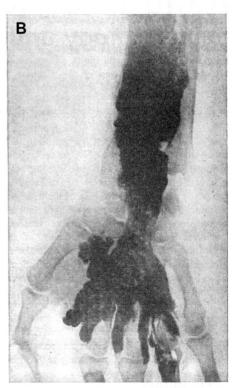

Fig. 1. (*A*) A radiographic plate published by Dr Kanavel, demonstrating the middle palmar space following plaster-of-Paris injection. (*B*) A subsequent high-pressure injection, demonstrating the ability of purulent infections to expand into adjacent compartments under pressure. (*Courtesy of* Galter Health Sciences Library & Learning Center, Northwestern University Feinberg School of Medicine, Chicago, IL, USA.)

characteristics of domestic animal bites, are more frequently reported. Most studies are published out of urban hospitals in large metropolitan areas. Patients treated in primary care facilities or in rural areas likely represent a large portion of injuries and often go unaccounted.

Incidence

Two-thirds of hand infections occur in men. Individuals of all ages are affected; the mean patient age is 40 years. More than one-third of hand infections are the result of trauma.[3] Domestic dog bites account for more than 800,000 health care visits in the United States annually. Cat bites are less common (estimated 400,000 per year in the United States) but more likely to cause infection; nearly half of all cat bites become infected without treatment.[4,5] Dogs have blunt teeth that leave an open wound that can drain, whereas cats' teeth penetrate and implant bacteria into deeper tissue. Two-thirds of pet bites affect the upper extremity.[6,7]

Postoperative surgical site infections are rare in hand surgery: 1.7 per 1000 procedures. Approximately 10% of patients with a surgical site infection require a secondary procedure.[8] Most infections are effectively treated with oral antibiotics.

Morbidity and Sequelae

Infections of the hand can lead to loss of function and disability, even when treated promptly. Infections of the flexor or extensor tendon spaces can lead to tendon necrosis, adhesions, and chronic stiffness. Intra-articular infections in the digits or carpus often cause progressive arthritis and require salvage procedures. Severe deep space infections and necrotizing fasciitis result in extensive soft tissue damage that sometimes requires flap coverage or amputation.

Microbiology and Antibacterial Resistance

Staphylococcus aureus, a round gram-positive bacteria, is the most common cause of hand infections.[9] In most areas of the United States, community-acquired methicillin-resistant *S aureus* (CA-MRSA) is the most common strain with culture rates approaching 50%.[10,11] *Beta-hemolytic streptococcus*, another round gram-positive bacteria, is the second most common cause of common hand infections. A causative organism cannot be identified in 1 of every 10 infections.[3]

Penicillin became available in 1929.[12] By 1955, more than 70% of *Staphylococcus* cultures were penicillin-resistant.[13] The rate of multidrug-resistant organisms has increased with the use of broad-spectrum antibiotics; 46% of *S aureus* strains are resistant to methicillin, 31% to clindamycin, and 56% to levofloxacin.[14]

Economic Impact

The cost of treating hand infections varies widely. A course of outpatient antibiotics is relatively inexpensive; however, surgery, maintenance of indwelling intravenous (IV) catheters, and IV treatments can be significantly more costly. In addition, many patients with hand infections are needlessly transferred to tertiary centers for care that can be provided at lower-level hospitals and clinics.[15] The cost of treating dog and cat bites ranges from $1880 to $82,000.[16] Little has been published on the cost of postoperative infections in hand surgery. A Veterans Affairs study found that patients who developed superficial surgical site infections incur a 1.25 times greater expense, whereas deep surgical site infections involving muscle or implants cost 1.93 times more.[17]

RISK FACTORS AND COMORBIDITIES

Although many hand infections result from trauma,[3] several risk factors predispose individuals to infection. This section presents common risk factors for upper extremity infection and their unique characteristics.

Diabetes

Type 2 diabetes mellitus is the most prevalent, modifiable, chronic illness in the United States. The Centers for Disease Control and Prevention (CDC) estimates that 30.3 million people are diabetic, 7.2 million of whom are undiagnosed.[18] Diabetes is a risk factor for several common hand conditions such as carpal tunnel syndrome and trigger finger.[19] Diabetic patients are at increased risk of idiopathic and postoperative infection, and are more likely to require operative intervention for infection.[20–22] Hand surgeons must have increased suspicion for atypical hand infections; fungi and rare species are more common in this population.[23]

Human Immunodeficiency Virus

More than 1 million adults are infected with human immunodeficiency virus (HIV) in the United States.[24] Patients with HIV have progressive failure of their immune system, which allows opportunistic infections to thrive. They have a higher rate of severe, necrotizing infection and more frequently require aggressive surgical debridement.[25,26]

Immunosuppression

Patients who are pharmacologically immunosuppressed for organ transplants, autoimmune disorders, and other medical conditions are at increased risk for infection. Deep space infection and osteomyelitis are far more common in these patients than in the general population.[27]

Hand surgeons often treat rheumatoid patients and must be knowledgeable on antirheumatic drugs. Traditional disease-modifying antirheumatic drugs (DMARDs), such as methotrexate, do not increase infection risk.[28] Patients may continue methotrexate in the perioperative period. Biologic DMARDs antagonize interleukin (IL)-1, IL-6, or tumor necrosis factor (TNF)-alpha. Anti-TNF-alpha medications increase the risk of skin and soft tissue infection in a dose-dependent manner.[29,30] Clinical guidelines for managing biologic DMARDs at the time of surgery do not yet exist. Patients, rheumatologists, and surgeons must work together to devise a medication plan based on individual needs and risks.

Intravenous Drug Use

It is estimated that 1 million people are active IV drug users (IVDU) in the United States.[31] IVDU is one of the strongest risk factors for CA-MRSA infection and necrotizing fasciitis.[32,33] Patients with poor vein access often turn to subcutaneous injection (known as "skin popping"), which has the highest risk of infection among drug administration methods.[34] Although a difficult patient population to treat, it is important to recognize and refer IVDUs to social work and addiction services in an attempt to reduce future health problems. Low-cost educational programs significantly reduce unsafe injecting practices and reduce injection site complications by 27% compared with controls.[35]

Occupation

Some professions predispose individuals to atypical infections. Examples include the following:

- Veterinarians and animal workers
  - *Pasteurella multocida*: An anaerobic, gram-negative coccobacilli that is part of the normal bacterial flora within the oropharynx of animals, most commonly domestic cats and dogs. It leads to purulent hand infections

after animal bites. Amoxicillin plus a beta-lactam inhibitor is the treatment of choice[36]

- Aquarists or fisherman
  - *Mycobacterium marinum*: Results in aquarium granuloma, an erythematous, nodule/s that can ulcerate as it matures. A history of working with aquariums or aquatic species, including shellfish, is common. Similar to tuberculosis, an extended course of multidrug antibacterial therapy is required for treatment[37] (**Fig. 2**).
- Horticulturists
  - *Sporothrix schenckii*: Sporotrichosis, commonly known as rose gardener's disease, is a fungal infection. It most commonly affects cutaneous tissue through direct inoculation when the skin is punctured by plant material (rose thorns, hay, sphagnum moss). Treatment is 3 to 6 months of itraconazole.[38]
- Dentists
  - *Herpes simplex virus*: Also known as Herpetic Whitlow, due to direct inoculation of the virus on the fingers. Presents as a painful finger with swelling and erythema and subsequent formation of clear fluid-filled vesicles. The disease is self-limiting, and surgical debridement is not

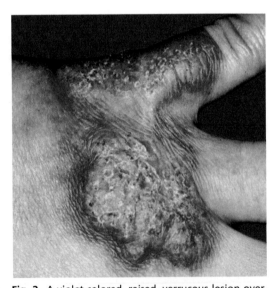

Fig. 2. A violet-colored, raised, verrucous lesion overlying the dorsal fourth and fifth metacarpophalangeal joints, demonstrating a typical appearance of Aquarium Granuloma. Cutaneous lesions surrounding joints as seen here can lead to stiffness and contracture. Surgical debridement may be necessary for large, necrotic wounds. (*From* Wu TS, Chiu CH, Yang CH, et al. Fish Tank Granuloma Caused by Mycobacterium marinum. PLoS One 2012; 7(7): e41296; with permission.)

recommended as it can disseminate the underlying infection.[39]

Regional

Globally, purulent hand infections are most commonly the result of *S aureus*; however, there are unique infections that are native to areas of Africa, Asia, and South America. Symptoms may manifest months to years after initial exposure, and even brief travel to endemic areas can predispose individuals. Travel history should be elicited in patients with atypical infections.

- Tuberculosis
  - Caused by *Mycobacterium tuberculosis*. In the upper extremity, the most common presentation is tenosynovitis, osteomyelitis, or deep space infection. Surgical debridement is often necessary and can reveal "rice bodies," as demonstrated in **Fig. 4**. The "rice bodies" are in fact outpouchings of synovial membrane that contain tuberculoid material[40] (**Fig. 3**).
- Buruli ulcer
  - The result of *Mycobacterium ulcerans*, an acid-fast bacteria. Up to 5000 people are affected globally per year, mostly in Central and West Africa, Australia, and tropical parts of South America. One-third of cases affect the upper extremity. Initial presentation is a benign and painless nodule or area of swelling that ulcerates within 3 to 4 weeks. Mycolactone, a toxin produced by *M ulcerans*, causes soft tissue destruction. Definitive diagnosis requires tissue culture but can take up to 8 weeks. Polymerase chain reaction testing exists for diagnosis but is commonly unavailable in endemic areas[41] (**Fig. 4**).
- Leishmaniasis
  - The result of one of more than a dozen known protozoa, the Leishmania family, subcategorized into New World versus Old World species. The disease is spread through the bites of sandflies and affects up to 1 million individuals per year. Cutaneous leishmaniasis is the most common form of the disease, which slowly develops over weeks to months after initial exposure. The lesions are usually raised papules or ulcerations, and are frequently painless[42] (**Fig. 5**).
- Yaws
  - A historically common cutaneous infection caused by *Treponema pallidum pertenue*. It is spread through direct contact and most commonly affects children. Yaws

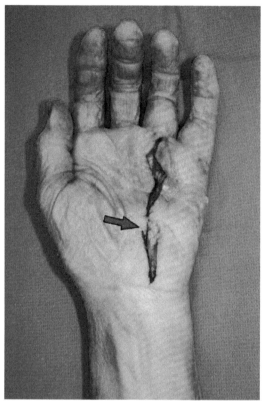

Fig. 3. Mycobacterial infection of the volar hand. The arrow demonstrates rice bodies exiting an incision decompressing the carpal tunnel and middle palmar space. Rice bodies can become space-occupying lesions within the carpal tunnel, leading to an acutely developing carpal tunnel syndrome.

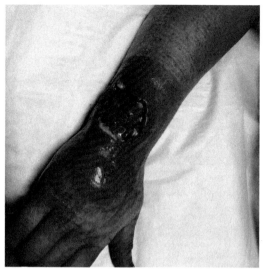

Fig. 4. A Buruli ulcer of the dorsal forearm and hand. Note the granular-appearing tissue at the base of the ulcer, suggesting a more chronic infection. Erythema extending distally into the dorsal hand from the large ulceration demonstrates the expanding nature of Buruli ulcers. Left untreated, Buruli ulcer in the hand and forearm can lead to extensor and flexor tendon disruption. (*From* Yerramilli A, Tay EL, Stewardson AJ, et al. The location of Australian Buruli ulcer lesions—Implications for unravelling disease transmission. PLoS Neglected Tropical Diseases 2017;11(8):e0005800; with permission.)

presents as a single "mother" papilloma that eventually expands into adjacent "daughter" lesions. Left untreated, the disease will progress to a secondary form, which causes diffuse raised yellow lesions on the extremities and can cause desquamation of the palms and feet. Surgery is rarely indicated, as treatment with a single dose of penicillin or azithromycin is successful in most cases[43] (**Fig. 6**).

DIAGNOSIS AND MANAGEMENT OF HAND INFECTIONS
Diagnosis

All encounters should begin with a complete medical history and hand examination. Clarify the mechanism of injury, duration of symptoms, and any treatment to date. Occupation, hobbies, and recent exposures may guide diagnosis. Tetanus vaccination status should be verified in any patient with an open trauma or bite injury. Tetanus

immunoglobulin and toxoid should be administered to patients who are not up to date on boosters.

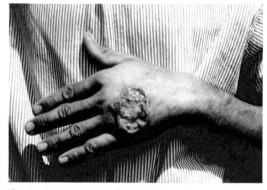

Fig. 5. Cutaneous Leishmaniasis resulting in a large dorsal hand lesion with deep central ulceration and hyperkeratotic, heaped and raised borders. Although wounds can be quite extensive, surgical debridement is often unnecessary, as the wounds frequently heal with medical management. (*Courtesy of* Centers for Disease Control and Prevention (CDC) and D.S. Martin.)

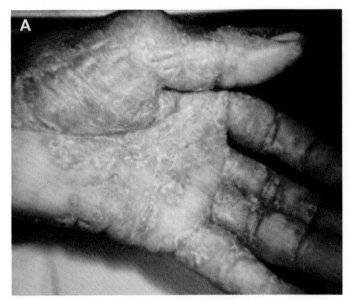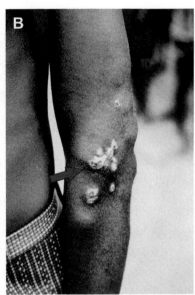

Fig. 6. (A) Loss of palmar epithelium is commonly seen in secondary and tertiary Yaws. (B) Yellow papillomas and ulcers of the proximal dorsal forearm; the arrow marks a likely "mother" lesion, with surrounding daughter lesions. Initially these lesions may be painless, but can become painful over time. (*Courtesy of* [A] Centers for Disease Control and Prevention (CDC) and S. Lindsley; and [B] Centers for Disease Control and Prevention (CDC) and P. Perine.)

An individual with MRSA who has not been exposed to a health care facility within the past year is assumed to have CA-MRSA. Making this distinction is important, as CA-MRSA is known to carry a unique gene sequence coding for Panton-Valentine leucocidin, a toxin that can increase local soft tissue damage.[44]

Infectious symptoms such as fevers and chills are often absent in patients with hand infections. Likewise, initial laboratory evaluation of white blood cell count, erythrocyte sedimentation rate, and C-reactive protein are frequently normal.[3] Diagnosis is largely clinical, based on the predictable presentations and patterns of infections.

Necrotizing fasciitis should be considered in all patients with rapid change in clinical examination. Progression of erythema, tense swelling (peau d'orange skin), and pain out of proportion with the examination should raise suspicion. Necrotizing fasciitis is a clinical diagnosis, but a basic metabolic panel and complete blood count are useful for calculating an LRINEC (Laboratory Risk Indicator for Necrotizing Fasciitis) score. A score greater than 6 has been shown to have a 92% positive predictive value and 96% negative predictive value[45] (**Table 1**).

Radiographs are obtained to rule out fracture and retained foreign bodies. Ultrasound can be helpful to diagnose fluid collections, radiolucent foreign bodies, and joint effusions.[46,47] MRI with and without contrast is valuable in diagnosis of deep space infection, foreign bodies, and differentiation between soft tissue edema versus fluid collections.

Management Principles

Purulent infections, such as felons, abscesses, and paronychia, are treated with debridement and antibiotics. When possible, cultures should be sent before antibiotics are given. Incisions should be placed directly over the area of maximum fluctuance and should be large enough for easy access to and complete drainage of the infection. Longitudinal incisions allow for extension proximally and distally if needed but should not cross flexion creases perpendicularly. All necrotic tissue must be debrided. Blunt dissection can be used to release areas of loculation. Wounds should be left open, packed with gauze to prevent premature closure, dressed at least daily, and examined frequently.

Because of increasing multidrug resistance, the CDC now recommends antibiotics with empiric MRSA coverage when local populations display MRSA growth/activity in more than 10% of cultures.[48] It is important to aggressively treat MRSA infections, as systemic dissemination of MRSA is associated with increased length of hospital stay, overall treatment cost, and mortality when compared with non–methicillin-resistant

Table 1
Laboratory risk indicator for necrotizing fasciitis (LR1NEC) score

Variable, Units	β	Score
C-reactive protein, mg/L		
<150	0	0
≥150	3.5	4
Total white cell count, per mm^3		
<15	0	0
15–25	05	1
>25	2.1	2
Hemoglobin, g/dL		
>13.5	0	0
11–135	0.6	1
<11	1.8	2
Sodium, mmol/L		
≥135	0	0
<135	1.8	2
Creatinine, μmol/L		
≤141	0	0
>141	1.8	2
Glucose, mmol/L		
≤10	0	0
>10	1.2	1

From Wong CH, Khin LW, Heng KS, et al. The LRINEC (Laboratory Risk Indicator for Necrotizing Fasciitis) score: a tool for distinguishing necrotizing fasciitis from other soft tissue infections. Crit Care Med 2004;32(7):1536; with permission.

species.[49,50] Antibiotic coverage should be narrowed based on culture sensitivity data. An extended course of intravenous antibiotic therapy is often required for deep space or recurrent infections, as well as osteomyelitis.

Rehabilitation

Soft dressings are preferred postoperatively. When immobilization is necessary, it should be discontinued as early as possible. The use of slings should be avoided, as they are unnecessary and cause shoulder and elbow stiffness. Occupational therapy is mandatory and should begin immediately to maximize hand function. Even with appropriate treatment and therapy, residual hand dysfunction is common after infections.

SUMMARY

Upper extremity infections encompass a wide variety of pathologic conditions and are a significant public health problem worldwide. A complete history and physical examination with special focus on known risk factors (medical comorbidities, drug use, occupation, and geography) is mandatory. Prompt treatment is required to prevent the long-term sequelae.

DISCLOSURE

The work was supported by a Midcareer Investigator Award in Patient-Oriented Research (2 K24-AR053120–06) to K.C. Chung. The content is solely the responsibility of the authors and does not necessarily represent the official views of the National Institutes of Health.

REFERENCES

1. Kanavel AB. An anatomical, experimental, and clinical study of acute phlegmons of the hand. Surg Gynecol Obstet 1905;1:221–60.
2. Kanavel AB. Infections of the hand. 1st edition. Philadelphia: Lea & Febiger; 1912.
3. Houshian S, Seyedipour S, Wedderkopp N. Epidemiology of bacterial hand infections. Int J Infect Dis 2006;10(4):315–9.
4. Elenbaas RM, McNabney WK, Robinson WA. Evaluation of prophylactic oxacillin in cat bite wounds. Ann Emerg Med 1984;13:155–7.
5. Kizer KW. Epidemiologic and clinical aspects of animal bite injuries. J Am Coll Emerg Phys 1979;8:134–41.
6. Weiss HB, Friedman DI, Coben JH. Incidence of dog bite injuries treated in emergency departments. JAMA 1998;279:51–3.
7. Goldstein EJ. Bite wounds and infection. Clin Infect Dis 1992;14:633–8.
8. Menendez ME, Lu N, Unizony S, et al. Surgical site infection in hand surgery. Int Orthop 2015;39(11):2191–8.
9. Florey ME, Williams RE. Hand infections treated with penicillin. Lancet 1944;1:73.
10. Kistler JM, Thoder JJ, Ilyas AM. MRSA incidence and antibiotic trend in urban hand infections: a 10-year lognitudinal study. Hand (N Y) 2019;14(4):449–54.
11. Imahara SD, Friedrich JB. Community-acquired methicillin-resistant *Staphylococcus aureus* in surgically treated hand infections. J Hand Surg Am 2010;35:97–103.
12. Fleming A. On antibacterial action of cultures of penicillium, with special reference to their use in isolating of *B. influenzae*. Br J Exp Pathol 1929;19:226.
13. Finland M. Emergency of antibiotic-resistant bacteria. N Engl J Med 1956;253:909.
14. Kistler JM, Vroome CM, Ramsey FV, et al. Increasing multidrug antibiotics resistance in MRSA infections

of the hand: a 10-year analysis of the risk factors. Hand (N Y) 2019. 1558944719837693.

15. Hartzell TL, Kuo P, Eberlin KR, et al. The overutilization of resources in patients with acute upper extremity trauma and infection. J Hand Surg Am 2013;38(4):766–73.

16. Benson LS, Edwards SL, Schiff AP, et al. Dog and cat bites to the hand: treatment and cost assessment. J Hand Surg Am 2006;31(3):468–73.

17. Schweizer ML, Cullen JJ, Perencevich EN, et al. Costs associated with surgical site infections in veterans affairs hospitals. JAMA Surg 2014;149(6):575–81.

18. Centers for Disease Control and Prevention. Prevalence of Both Diagnosed and Undiagnosed Diabetes. 2018. Available at: https://www.cdc.gov/diabetes/data/statistics-report/diagnosed-undiagnosed.html. Accessed April 13, 2019.

19. Perkins BA, Olaleye D, Bril V. Carpal tunnel syndrome in patients with diabetic polyneuropathy. Diabetes Care 2002;25:565–9.

20. Wener BC, Teran VA, Cancienne J, et al. The association of perioperative glycemic control with postoperative surgical site infection following open carpal tunnel release in patients with diabetes. Hand (N Y) 2019;14(3):324–32.

21. Sharma K, Pan D, Friedman J, et al. Quantifying the effect of diabetes on surgical hand and forearm infections. J Hand Surg Am 2018;43(2):105–14.

22. Gonzalez MH, Bochar S, Novotny J, et al. Upper extremity infections in patient with diabetes mellitus. J Hand Surg Am 1992;24(4):682–6.

23. Jalil A, Barlaan PI, Fung BK, et al. Hand infection in diabetic patients. Hand Surg 2011;16(3):307–12.

24. Centers for Disease Control and Prevention. HIV in the United States and Dependent Areas. Available at: https://www.cdc.gov/hiv/statistics/overview/ataglance.html. Accessed April 13, 2019.

25. Gonzalez M, Nikoleit J, Weinzweig N, et al. Upper extremity infections in patient with the human immunodeficiency virus. J Hand Surg 1998;23(2):348–52.

26. McAuliffe JA, Seltzer DG, Hornicek F. Upper-extremity infections in patients seropositive for human immunodeficiency virus. J Hand Surg 1997;22A:1084–90.

27. Klein MB, Chang J. Management of hand and upper-extremity infections in heart transplant recipients. Plast Reconstr Surg 2000;106(3):598–601.

28. Jain A, Witbreuk M, Ball C, et al. Influence of steroids and methotrexate on wound complications after elective rheumatoid hand and wrist surgery. J Hand Surg Am 2002;27(3):449–55.

29. Dixon WG, Watson K, Lunt M, et al. Rates of serious infection, including site-specific and bacterial intracellular infection, in rheumatoid arthritis patients receiving anti-tumor necrosis factor therapy: results from the British Society for Rheumatology Biologics Register. Arthritis Rheum 2006;54(8):2368–76.

30. Singh JA, Cameron C, Noorbaloochi S, et al. Risk of serious infection in biological treatment of patients with rheumatoid arthritis: a systematic review and meta-analysis. Lancet 2015;386(9990):258–65.

31. Lansky A, Finlayson T, Johnson C, et al. Estimating the number of persons who inject drugs in the United States by meta-analysis to calculate national rates of HIV and hepatitis C virus infections. PLoS One 2014;9:e97596.

32. Nourbakhsh A, Papafragkou S, Dever LL, et al. Stratification of the risk factors of community-acquired methicillin-resistant *Staphylococcus aureus* hand infection. J Hand Surg Am 2010;35(7):1135–41.

33. Sunderland IR, Friedrich JB. Predictors of mortality and limb loss in necrotizing soft tissue infections of the upper extremity. J Hand Surg Am 2009;32:1900–1.

34. Thomas WO III, Almand JD, Stark GB, et al. Hand infections secondary to subcutaneous illicit drug injection. Ann Plast Surg 1995;34:27–31.

35. Roux P, Le Gall JM, Debrus M, et al. Innovative community-based educational face-to-face intervention to reduce HIV, hepatitis C virus and other blood-borne infectious risks in difficult-to-reach people who inject drugs: results from the ANRS-AERLI intervention study. Addiction 2016;111(1):94–106.

36. Wilkie IW, Harper M, Boyce JD, et al. *Pasteurella multocida*: diseases and pathogenesis. Curr Top Microbiol Immunol 2012;361:1–22.

37. Wu TS, Chiu CH, Yang CH, et al. Fish tank granuloma caused by *Mycobacterium marinum*. PLoS One 2012;7(7):e41296.

38. Barros MBL, Paes RA, Schubach AO. *Sporothrix schenckii* and sporotrichosi. Clin Microbiol Rev 2011;24(4):633–54.

39. Haedicke GJ, Grossman JA, Fisher AE. Herpetic whitlow of the digits. J Hand Surg Br 1989;14:443–6.

40. Al-Qattan MM, Al-Namla A, Al-Thunayan A, et al. Tuberculosis of the hand. J Hand Surg Am 2011;36(A):1413–22.

41. Loftus MJ, Tay EL, Globan M, et al. Epidemiology of buruli ulcer infections, Victoria, Australia, 2011-2016. Emerg Infect Dis 2018;24(11):1988–97.

42. Torres-Guerrero E, Quintanilla-Cedillo MR, Ruiz-Esmenjaud J, et al. Leishmaniasis: a review. F1000Res 2017;6:750.

43. Kazadi WM, Asiedu KB, Agana N, et al. Epidemiology of yaws: an update. Clin Epidemiol 2014;6:119–28.

44. O'Malley M, Fowler J, Ilyas AM. Community-acquired methicillin-resistant *Staphylococcus aureus* infection of the hand: prevalence and timeliness of treatment. J Hand Surg Am 2009;34(3):504–8.

45. Wong CH, Khin LW, Heng KS, et al. The LRINEC (Laboratory Risk Indicator for Necrotizing Fasciitis)

score: a tool for distinguishing necrotizing fasciitis from other soft tissue infections. Crit Care Med 2004;32(7):1535–41.

46. Marvel BA, Budhram GR. Bedside ultrasound in the diagnosis of complex hand infections: a case series. J Emerg Med 2015;48(1):63–8.

47. Gottlieb J, Mailhot T, Chilstrom M. Point-of-care ultrasound diagnosis of deep space hand infection. J Emerg Med 2016;50(3):458–61.

48. Gorwitz RJ, Jernigan DB, Powers JH, et al. Centers for Disease Control and Prevention-Convened Experts' Meeting on Management of MRSA in the Community. Strategies for clinical management of MRSA in the community: Summary of an Experts' Meeting Convened by the Centers for Disease Control and Prevention. Available at: http://www.cdc.gov/mrsa/pdf/MRSA-Strategies-ExpMtg Summary-2006.pdf. Accessed April 28, 2019.

49. Resch A, Wilke M, Fink C. The cost of resistance: incremental cost of methicillin-resistant staphylococcus aureus (MRSA) in German hospitals. Eur J Health Econ 2009;10:287–97.

50. Lodise TP, McKinnon PS. Clinical and economic impact of methicillin resistance in patients with Staphylococcus aureus bacteremia. Diagn Microbiol Infect Dis 2005;52(2):113–22.

Imaging and Laboratory Workup for Hand Infections

Colin M. Whitaker, MD[a], Sara Low, MD[a], Tetyana Gorbachova, MD[b],
James S. Raphael, MD[c], Chris Williamson, MD[d],*

KEYWORDS

- Hand infections • MRI • CT • Ultrasound • ESR • CRP

KEY POINTS

- Hand and upper-extremity infections are usually a clinical diagnosis.
- Computed tomographic scans are sensitive in detecting gas in the soft tissues and provide the most detailed evaluation of bony anatomy.
- MRI is useful for evaluating the extent of infection in both soft tissue and bone marrow.
- The addition of contrast improves diagnostic accuracy in detecting abscesses and infection.
- Laboratory values are helpful in supporting the diagnosis of infection but are less specific; baseline white blood cell count, erythrocyte sedimentation rate, and C-reactive protein levels are recommended and generally used to trend disease progression.

INTRODUCTION

Hand infections are frequently seen by primary care, emergency, and orthopedic providers and can afflict all communities.[1,2] Accurate and prompt diagnosis and treatment of hand and upper-extremity infections are imperative in order to reduce morbidity related to stiffness and decreased function.[2,3]

Typically, hand infections can be diagnosed clinically. However, because of the complex anatomy of the hand and varying degrees of presentation, diagnosis is not always straightforward. Both imaging and laboratory evaluation aid in diagnosis. Commonly used imaging modalities, radiography, ultrasound (US), computed tomography (CT), and MRI, are addressed in later discussion. Nuclear medicine imaging techniques, such as bone scintigraphy, have been largely replaced by CT and MRI in the diagnosis of hand infection, but can be used in certain scenarios.

X-ray technology was first described by William Conrad Röntgen in 1895.[4] In the present day, radiography is recommended as a first line of imaging for almost all forms of hand infections. High spatial resolution of radiography enables visualization of fine details of cortical bone, which, in the setting of infection, is critical for detection of focal demineralization, periosteal reaction, cortical erosions, and associated fractures (**Fig. 1**). Radiographic depiction of erosions and soft tissue calcifications provides important differential diagnosis of noninfectious mimickers, such as gout or calcific tendinitis (**Fig. 2**). Beyond detection of calcifications, gas, and radiopaque foreign bodies, the role of

[a] Department of Orthopedic Surgery, Einstein Healthcare Network, 1200 West Tabor Road, Willowcrest Building, 4th Floor, Philadelphia, PA 19141, USA; [b] Musculoskeletal Imaging, Department of Radiology, Einstein Healthcare Network, Jefferson Medical College, 5501 Old York Road, Philadelphia, PA 19141, USA; [c] Einstein Healthcare Network, 1200 West Tabor Road, Willowcrest Building, 4th Floor, Philadelphia, PA 19141, USA; [d] Hand and Upper Extremity Division, Einstein Healthcare Network, Department of Orthopedic Surgery, 170 West Germantown Pike, Suite C-1, East Norriton, PA 19401, USA
* Corresponding author.
E-mail address: cwilliamsonmd@gmail.com

Hand Clin 36 (2020) 285–299
https://doi.org/10.1016/j.hcl.2020.03.002
0749-0712/20/© 2020 Elsevier Inc. All rights reserved.

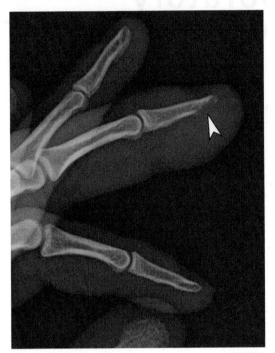

Fig. 1. Felon in a 24-year-old man after sustaining a small laceration 2 weeks before. Lateral radiograph of the hand demonstrates soft tissue swelling over the long finger, cortical resorption, and focal erosion (*arrowhead*) at the volar aspect of the tuft consistent with osteomyelitis.

radiographs is limited in the evaluation of soft tissues and bone marrow.

Cross-sectional imaging modalities, such as CT or MRI, can provide assessment of compartmental anatomy and detect a spectrum of soft tissue abnormalities as well as acute osteomyelitis. Since the advent of CT in 1973, the technology has advanced rapidly, acquiring up to 1200 sections per second.[5] From the 1970s through the early 2000s, the development of multidetector CT technology and multiplanar reformation has allowed 3-dimensional spatial resolution[5,6] (**Fig. 3**). Dual-energy CT is a promising new technique that provides additional information about tissue composition based on differences in in x-ray attenuation at 2 different energy levels.[7]

MRI technology followed closely on the heels of CT technology and was adapted into common clinical use in 1984, 6 years after Dr John Belliveau's successful experiments.[8] It provides superior contrast resolution compared with CT. MRI depicts contrast between various tissues in the body based on differences in their proton resonance when the patient is placed in a strong external magnetic field, and the area of interest is interrogated by applying radiofrequency pulses

and gradient coils. Because the hand is relatively small and contains numerous complex structures in close proximity to each other, adequate spatial and contrast resolution is required for proper evaluation. Technical advances, such as hand and upper-extremity dedicated surface coils and high-field-strength magnets, have substantially improved the resolution of hand MRIs.[9–11] Compared with 1.5 T, higher main magnetic field strength of 3.0 T allows 1.6 to 2.6 times increase in contrast to noise ratio between the various structures of the hand, advancing the diagnostic capability of MRI by improving image quality and decreasing scan time.[9,10,12]

Typical MR imaging protocol uses a combination of T1 and so-called fluid-sensitive sequences, which include short tau inversion recovery (STIR), fat-suppressed T2-weighted, and proton density (PD) weighted images.

- Fluid-sensitive sequences: accentuate appearance of fluid and edema, which is present in most pathologic conditions of the bone and soft tissue
- T1-weighted images: provide evaluation of anatomy and accurately depict fatty tissue, which adds specificity in diagnosis of bone and soft tissue infection

In both CT and MRI, the use of intravenous (IV) contrast improves diagnostic accuracy of detection of abscesses, sinus tracts, and necrotic tissue.

US offers several advantages because it can be performed at the bedside, in patients who may have contraindications to MRI, and does not have the radiation risk associated with CT scans, all while being less costly.[13] US is very sensitive in the detection of fluid collections. It allows assessment of vascular flow (**Fig. 4**), visualization of nonradiopaque foreign bodies, as well as dynamic evaluation of the tendons and real-time guidance for percutaneous interventions. Among several technical factors, the diagnostic utility of US is operator dependent and relies on focused examination tailored to a specific clinical question and area of interest.[14]

Laboratory values are also helpful in the diagnosis of hand infections but are less specific and should be used in conjunction with clinical examination. In general, C-reactive protein (CRP) and erythrocyte sedimentation rate (ESR) are commonly obtained in cases of infection (**Table 1**).

Because ESR and CRP levels are increased in states of inflammation and are not specific to infection, their use is often supportive and limited

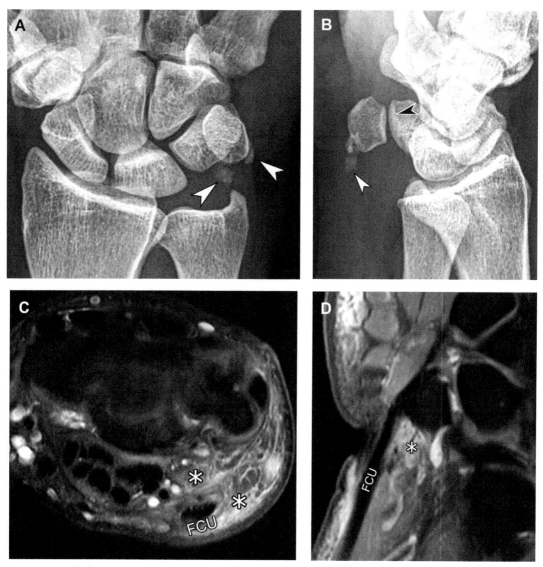

Fig. 2. Acute calcific tendinitis in a 42-year-old man with pain, swelling, and redness over the volar ulnar aspect of the wrist. (*A*) Posterioanterior (PA) and (*B*) external oblique radiographs of the wrist demonstrate characteristic cloudlike soft tissue calcifications (*arrowheads*) near pisiform (P) along expected insertion of flexor carpi ulnaris tendon (FCU). (*C*) Axial T2-weighted fat-suppressed MRI and (*D*) sagittal PD weighted fat-suppressed image depict nonspecific soft tissue swelling (*asterisks*) subcutaneously and deep to FCU tendon. Calcifications are frequently inconspicuous on MRI.

to monitoring progression or resolution of infection.[15] Immunosuppressed patients may also have normal ESR/CRP levels because of the inability to mount an immune response.[18] Recent interest has emerged in additional markers, such as interleukin-6 (IL-6) and procalcitonin. Although IL-6 has been studied and found to be consistent with orthopedic periprosthetic joint infections, procalcitonin has been extensively studied in medical literature and shown to be elevated in bacterial infections.[19,20]

CELLULITIS

Cellulitis, an infection of the skin and subcutaneous tissue, presents with erythema, swelling, and pain. The diagnosis is often complicated by the fact that a multitude of other hand infections and noninfectious conditions can also have similar overlying skin changes. Radiographic signs of cellulitis include skin thickening, soft tissue swelling, and obliteration of fat planes.[21] US can be useful in the diagnosis of cellulitis. Thickened

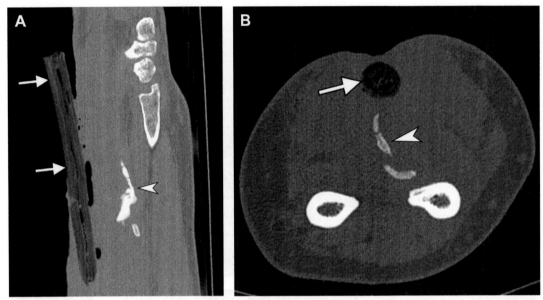

Fig. 3. Foreign body in a 47-year-old male psychiatric patient with repeated self-inflicted wounds in the left volar forearm. (*A*) Unenhanced sagittal reformatted CT image and (*B*) axial CT image demonstrate large foreign body with air densities (*arrows in A, B*), a wooden stick, in the volar forearm, loss of soft tissue fat planes, and mature heterotopic ossification (*arrowhead*) related to multiple previous infections and debridement.

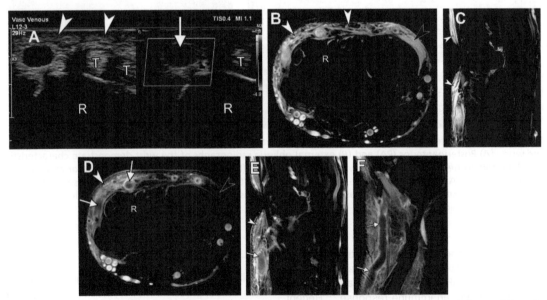

Fig. 4. Cellulitis and septic thrombophlebitis in a 30-year-old man. (*A*) Doppler US image shows edema of the subcutaneous fat (*arrowheads*) and absence of color flow in a thrombosed superficial vein (*arrow*) at the dorsum of the wrist (T, extensor tendons; R, radius). (*B*) Axial T2-weighted fat-suppressed image and (*C*) sagittal PD weighted fat-suppressed image demonstrate subcutaneous edema (*white arrowheads*) with confluent regions of fluid signal (*black arrowhead*) concerning for abscess. (*D*) Contrast-enhanced axial and (*E, F*) sagittal T1-weighted fat-suppressed images depict ill-defined reticular enhancement of the subcutaneous fat (*white arrowhead*), without rim-enhancing collections (*black arrowhead*), and thrombosed superficial veins (*arrows*) with enhancing walls consistent with thrombophlebitis.

Table 1 Comparison of commonly used inflammatory markers	
CRP	ESR
Direct indicator of the acute phase reaction Synthesized in the liver	Surrogate marker
Response to inflammatory mediators (ie, IL-6, IL-1, transforming growth factor-β, TNF-α)	Dependent on fibrinogen levels
Rises within 4–6 h of the inflammatory reaction Peaks at 36–50 h	Can take up to 48 h to increase
Returns to baseline 3–7 d (after initiation of treatment)	Normalizes over several weeks
Can be affected by hormone therapy, smoking, depression, chronic fatigue, cardiac ischemia	Influenced by several baseline conditions (ie, age, gender, anemia, pregnancy, chronic kidney disease, diabetes, malignancy)

Data from Refs.[15–17]

and abnormally hyperechoic skin and subcutaneous tissue can be appreciated. The subcutaneous tissue is classically described as "cobblestone," representing inflammatory exudate dissecting the tissues[22] (**Fig. 5**). However, this appearance is not specific to infection and can be appreciated in patients with subcutaneous edema because of venous or lymphatic stasis.[14] Color or power Doppler imaging can depict hyperemia seen with cellulitis, helping to differentiate it from noninfectious causes of edema.[13,23,24]

Cross-sectional imaging can be used to confirm cellulitis but is primarily used to exclude other disease processes (see **Fig. 5**). Similar to US, infectious and noninfectious causes of subcutaneous edema have a similar appearance on CT and MRI (**Fig. 6**). MRI findings of cellulitis include thickening of the subcutaneous tissues and linear or ill-defined increased signal intensity of superficial soft tissue on fluid-sensitive sequences (see **Fig. 4**), and corresponding low-signal intensity on T1-weighted images.[23,25] Focal fluid collections are not present in uncomplicated cellulitis, and no abnormal signal intensity should be seen in the underlying muscle.[26] Confluent edema may mask small collections on

unenhanced MRI, and administration of IV contrast may be required in such cases to detect abscesses.

ABSCESSES

An abscess is a collection of purulent material in a confined, localized space that often presents with diffuse hand swelling.[27,28] Radiographs can help exclude foreign bodies and associated fracture, but isolated abscesses typically appear as nonspecific soft tissue masses (**Fig. 7**A).

On US, an abscess is usually seen as a hypoechoic fluid collection.[22] It can occasionally be mobilized with the transducer and may vary in appearance as heterogeneously isoechoic or hyperechoic.[23] Color Doppler US will demonstrate surrounding hyperemia without vascular flow inside the collection[29] (**Fig. 7**). Absence of increased vascularity around a fluid collection makes it less likely to represent an inflammatory or infectious process.[24]

Several studies have demonstrated the benefit of US, especially in the emergency room (ER) setting. In 1 recent study, US had 96.7% sensitivity for abscess.[30] It has also been shown to impact management in almost half of cases when results were correlated with clinical findings.[31] The use of a water bath can be beneficial both for patient comfort and for improving image quality.[14]

On MRI, abscesses frequently appear as regions of confluent high-signal intensity on fluid-sensitive sequences, and corresponding intermediate to low signal replacing normal subcutaneous fat signal on T1-weighted images[32] (**Fig. 8**). Adjacent inflammation is typically present and may lead to overestimation of the abscess.[33] IV contrast can delineate abscesses showing peripheral rim enhancement and nonenhancing fluid and necrotic contents, which adds specificity in differentiating it from phlegmonous changes.[32,34] MRI is reported to be 89% sensitive and 80% specific for diagnosis of soft tissue abscess.[32]

CT can also be valuable when evaluating for abscesses. This scenario is especially true when US evaluation is technically difficult, for example, when obtaining an acoustic window is challenging because of an open wound or surgical dressing, or access to MRI is limited. CT can show retained radiopaque and some nonradiopaque foreign bodies (see **Fig. 3**). Muscle edema may also be present as well as intraabscess gas.[33] On CT, abscesses appear as fluid collection with variable internal attenuation, irregular margins, and a thick wall that enhances with IV contrast[33] (see **Fig. 8**).

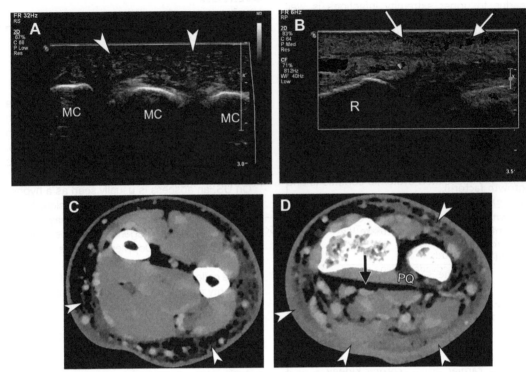

Fig. 5. (*A, B*) Cellulitis. Grayscale and color Doppler US images of the dorsum of the hand and wrist (metacarpal bones, MC; radius, R) of a 62-year-old diabetic woman show subcutaneous edema with cobblestone appearance (*arrowheads*) and hyperemia (*arrows*). Axial contrast-enhanced CT images of the wrist in a 47-year-old man demonstrate skin thickening, linear and diffuse subcutaneous edema (*arrowheads, C*). Note normal fat (*arrow, D*) in potential space of Parona overlying pronator quadratus (PQ) fascia.

SEPTIC ARTHRITIS

Septic arthritis is characterized by purulent exudate within the closed confines of a joint.[18]

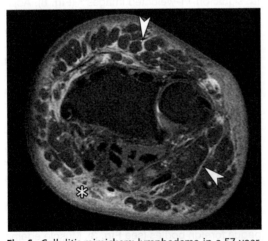

Fig. 6. Cellulitis mimickers: lymphedema in a 57-year-old woman with remote history of axial node dissection. Axial PD fat-suppressed image of the right wrist demonstrates prominent circumferential skin thickening and subcutaneous edema in diffuse (*asterisk*) and reticular (*arrowheads*) patterns.

Most patients present with a warm, red, and swollen joint. A thorough history taking is essential to rule out inflammatory causes, such as gout, pseudogout, lupus, or rheumatoid arthritis.

Blood cultures should be routinely obtained, particularly in patients presenting with systemic symptoms. Although the white blood cell (WBC) count is only elevated in about 50% of affected patients, ESR and CRP levels are reliably above normal.[18] Serum procalcitonin levels are 85.2% sensitive and 87.3% specific using a cutoff value of 0.4 ng/mL for septic arthritis and osteomyelitis.[35]

A positive joint fluid culture is considered the gold standard but lacks sensitivity.[35] Fluid analysis, including cell count and crystals review, should be performed. Historically, a cell count of 50,000 (75% polymorphonuclear leukocytes and glucose of 40 mg% less than fasting blood glucose level) is considered a septic joint.[18] Li and colleagues[36] suggested lowering the cell count threshold to 17,500, which correspondingly increased the sensitivity of the diagnosis of septic arthritis to 83% but led to a specificity of 67%.

In addition, Lenski and Scherer[37]'s evaluated synovial lactate levels and found it to have excellent

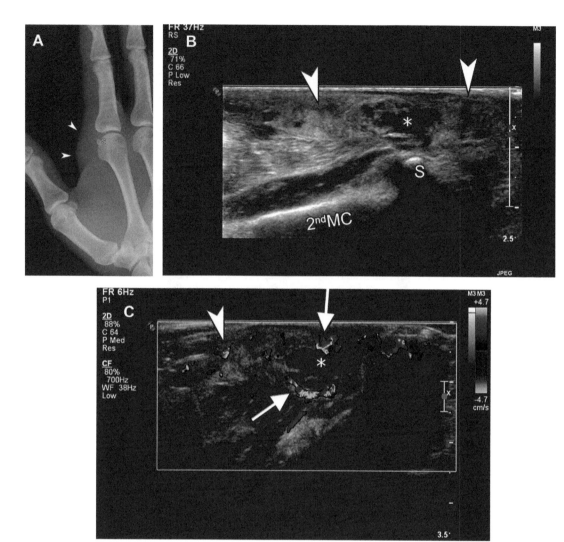

Fig. 7. Abscess and cellulitis in a 45-year-old diabetic woman. Oblique radiograph of the hand (A) demonstrates focal soft tissue swelling (*arrowheads*) over the radial sesamoid (S) of the second metacarpophalangeal (MCP) joint. (*B*) Grayscale and (*C*) color Doppler US images show diffusely thick echogenic soft tissues (*arrowheads*, *B*) with hyperemia (*arrowheads*, *C*), and a complex hypoechoic collection (*asterisk*) with echogenic rim that demonstrates increased color Doppler flow (*arrows*) consistent with abscess.

diagnostic potential to differentiate septic arthritis from gouty arthritis. Synovial lactate levels greater than 10 mmol/L were consistent with a diagnosis of septic arthritis, whereas levels lower than 4.3 mmol/L make it very unlikely.

Radiographs may be negative initially, but also may show joint capsule distention, periarticular soft tissue swelling, and juxtaarticular osteopenia.[38] Gas within the soft tissue or joint may indicate an anaerobic infection, but is also seen in penetrating injuries even without infection. Later in the course of the disease, uniform joint space narrowing secondary to cartilage destruction and osseous erosions can be appreciated[18] (**Figs. 9**

and **10**). In contradistinction to infection, osteoarthritis is typically associated with a nonuniform joint space loss, subchondral sclerosis, and osteophyte formation.[38] Acute gout may mimic infection clinically, and awareness of its classic radiographic features is critical for diagnosis (**Fig. 11**).

MRI features of septic arthritis include effusion, synovitis, periarticular soft tissue edema, abscess formation, and periarticular bone edema[39] (see **Fig. 9**). Graif and colleagues[40] found that bone erosions with marrow edema in the presence of synovial thickening and soft tissue edema were highly suggestive of septic arthritis, compared with the nonseptic joint.

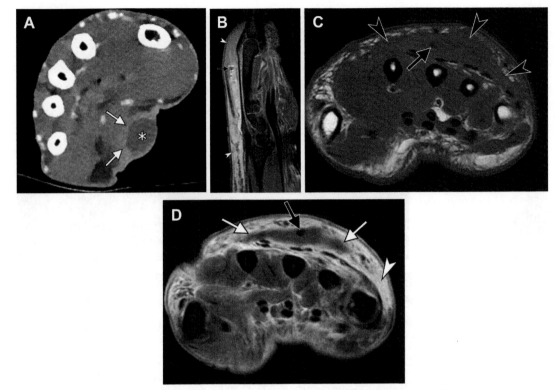

Fig. 8. Abscess. (*A*) Contrast-enhanced axial CT image of the hand in 39-year-old man with polysubstance abuse shows superficial fluid collection (*asterisk*) with thick peripheral enhancement (*arrows*) at the palmar aspect of the hand. (*B*) Sagittal PD weighted fat-suppressed image of the hand in a 66-year-old diabetic woman depicts dorsal soft tissue swelling (*arrowheads*) with focus of susceptibility artifact from gas bubble (*black arrow; B–D*). (*C*) Axial T1-weighted image shows confluent area of loss of normal subcutaneous fat (*arrowheads; C*) corresponding to a rim-enhancement collection on contrast-enhanced T1-weighted fat-suppressed image (*white arrows; D*). Contrast-enhanced images help differentiate collection from surrounding inflammatory changes (*arrowhead; D*).

OSTEOMYELITIS

Osteomyelitis is an infection of the bone and bone marrow.[41] ESR and CRP levels are almost always elevated in acute osteomyelitis, whereas they are elevated in only 65% of chronic osteomyelitis.[41–43] Hence, ESR and CRP levels have no correlation with final clinical outcome and are more commonly used for monitoring therapeutic efficacy.[41,43,44] In 1 study, ESR greater than 20 mm/h was associated with osteomyelitis recurrence.[45] In addition, WBC count rarely increases to greater than 15,000/mm^3 and can be normal in chronic osteomyelitis.[42] A positive microbiological culture, either from blood or from the affected bone, is essential to the diagnosis.[42]

Normal serum levels of procalcitonin are very low, less than 0.1 ng/mL (half-life 22–29 hours), and increase rapidly in response to bacterial endotoxin.[17,35] In a study of 82 patients, procalcitonin cutoff of 0.4 ng/mL was 65% to 85.2% sensitive

and 87.3% to 100% specific for diagnosing septic arthritis and osteomyelitis.[35] Other studies that used a cutoff of 0.2 to 0.3 ng/mL had a pooled sensitivity and specificity of 90% and 87%, respectively.[46] The use of procalcitonin in upper-extremity osteomyelitis has yet to become common practice, because there is a lack of osteomyelitis-specific literature.[17,46] IL-6 and tumor necrosis factor-alpha (TNF-α) have also been described to be associated with infection, such as bacterial osteomyelitis, peaking at greater than 200 pg/mL and greater than 100 pg/mL, respectively.[47]

Radiographs do not demonstrate changes in early acute osteomyelitis until up to 1 to 3 weeks following its onset.[33,41–43] Radiographic features include soft tissue swelling, haziness and loss of density of the affected bone, permeative pattern of bone destruction, cortical erosions, periostitis (**Fig. 12**) and, in some cases, osteosclerosis.[23,33,42] Gross destructive changes occur later

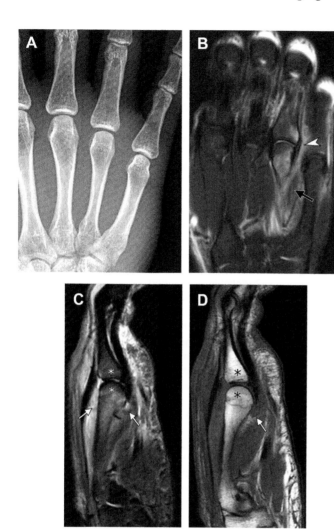

Fig. 9. Septic arthritis in a 24-year-old man after injecting drugs into the dorsal hand 1 week before. (*A*) PA radiograph of the hand demonstrates no abnormality. (*B*) Coronal sagittal PD weighted fat-suppressed image shows periarticular soft tissue swelling (*arrowhead*), bone marrow edema at both sides of the fourth MCP joint, and edema of adjacent intrinsic muscles (*arrow*). (*C*) Sagittal STIR and (*D*) T1-weighted images of the fourth MCP joint demonstrate complex joint effusion (*arrows*; *C, D*) associated with periarticular marrow edema (*asterisks*; *C*). Preserved normal fatty marrow signal (*asterisks*; *D*) indicates absence of osteomyelitis.

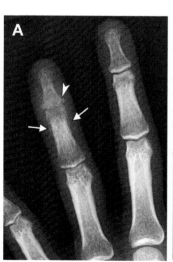
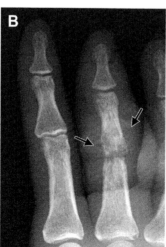

Fig. 10. (*A*) Septic arthritis and osteomyelitis of the fourth distal interphalangeal joint in a 32-year-old man with periarticular osteopenia, diffuse loss of joint space, and central erosions (*arrowhead*); periosteal reaction along the middle phalanx (*arrows*) indicates osteomyelitis. (*B*) In a 48-year-old homeless man, advanced osseous destruction is seen in the third proximal interphalangeal joint with soft tissue gas (*arrows*).

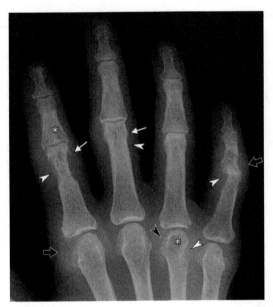

Fig. 11. Infection mimickers: gout in a 69-year-old man with acute hand pain and swelling. PA radiograph of the right hand demonstrates lobulated soft tissue swelling with increased radiodensity (*black arrows*) corresponding to tophi. There are multiple juxtaarticular erosions (*white arrowheads*), some demonstrating overhanging edges (*white arrows*) characteristic of gout. Note intraosseous erosions (*asterisk*) as well as preerosive changes with loss of white cortical line (*black arrowhead*). In contradistinction to infection, the joint spaces are preserved.

in the disease process.[42] Sequestrum and involucrum, which are sclerotic dense dead bone and reactive new bone formation around dead bone, respectively, are signs of chronic active osteomyelitis.[23,42] Sequestrum appears radiographically dense because it is devascularized and cannot undergo regional osteoporosis.[33]

CT studies provide improved evaluation of bony changes, such as cortical erosion, sequestrum, involucrum, and intraosseous fistulae.[33,41,42] Three-dimensional localization of sequestra facilitates surgical planning for complete removal, which is paramount to treatment success.[23]

MRI scans are currently the gold standard for diagnosing osteomyelitis and have a reported sensitivity of 82% to 100% for early osteomyelitis.[23,33] On T1-weighted images, areas of bone infected with osteomyelitis will appear hypointense, because the infection replaces normal fatty marrow signal[23,33] (see **Fig. 12**). On fluid-sensitive sequences, osteomyelitis is hyperintense, reflecting marrow edema.[23,33,42] Bone marrow hyperintensity on fluid-sensitive images without corresponding hypointensity on T1-weighted

images may suggest reactive marrow edema without osteomyelitis.[23] MRI may show periosteal elevation caused by subperiosteal collection of infectious material.[11] As cortical destruction occurs, MRI and CT scans may show focal irregularity of the cortex, with CT being superior in imaging of cortical bone detail.[11] Next, fluid-sensitive sequences may show a hyperintense linear signal within hypointense cortex, representing decompression of purulent material from bone into the surrounding soft tissues. Ultimately, this may form a sinus track to skin.[11] Osteomyelitis is also readily apparent as a hyperintense area on post–gadolinium-enhanced images.[33] However, if there is severely decreased blood supply secondary to high marrow pressure or bone necrosis, enhancement may not be present.[33]

Gadolinium-enhanced MRI may help differentiate active infection from postoperative fibrovascular scar.[42] Osteomyelitis is not uncommon at the site of orthopedic hardware, and metal artifact reduction sequences techniques have been developed to reduce image distortion from hardware.[48] Another caveat of MRI in osteomyelitis is that very young children who have a more hematopoietic and less fatty marrow may have less obvious hypointense signal on T1-weighted sequences.[33] Finally, MRI can overestimate the disease burden secondary to reactive marrow edema.[33,41]

Another described method of diagnosing early osteomyelitis that is more sensitive than radiography or CT is a nuclear bone scan or bone scintigraphy.[23,33] Technetium 99m (99mTc) methylene diphosphonate, which binds to sites of bony turnover, is the most common radiopharmaceutical used.[49] Osteomyelitis is seen on 3-phase bone scintigraphy as focal hyperperfusion, hyperemia, and increased uptake, particularly on the delayed images.[23,33] Essentially, if bone scintigraphy is negative, active infection can be excluded except in the case of marked bone marrow hypoperfusion.[23,33] The advantage of bone scans is whole-body imaging; however, bone scans can have false positives around sites of fracture, orthopedic hardware, or osteoarthritis.[23] As such, indium 111–labeled or 99mTc-labeled WBCs can be used to counter the limitation by metal artifact of MRI, CT, and regular bone scintigraphy.[23,33,42] PET with 2-[fluorine-18] fluoro-2-deoxy-D-glucose, performed alone or with CT, has great diagnostic utility and is sometimes interchangeable with bone scintigraphy, but is very costly.[23,41,49]

PYOGENIC TENOSYNOVITIS

Pyogenic flexor tenosynovitis (FTS) is a closed space infection of the flexor tendon sheath,

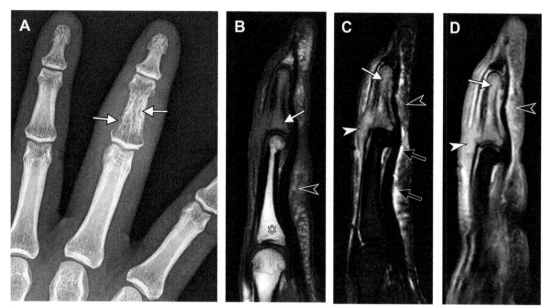

Fig. 12. Osteomyelitis in a 46-year-old man, who sustained a laceration 10 days ago. (*A*) PA radiograph demonstrates soft tissue swelling and permeative pattern of bone destruction with loss of bone density and tiny radiolucencies in the long finger middle phalanx (*arrows*). (*B*) Sagittal T1-weighted, (*C*) fat-suppressed T2-weighted, (*D*) and contrast-enhanced fat-suppressed T1-weighted sequences through the long finger demonstrate osteomyelitis with bone marrow edema (*arrow; C*) and replacement of normal medullary fat signal intensity throughout the middle phalanx (*arrow; B*), and corresponding enhancement (*arrow; D*), compared with normal signal in the proximal phalanx (*asterisk*). Note phlegmonous changes dorsally with diffuse enhancement (*white arrowheads; C, D*), surrounding cellulitis (*black arrowheads; B–D*), and FTS (*black arrows; B*).

between the visceral epitenon layer and outer parietal layer.[2,3] Laboratory values, such as WBC, ESR, and CRP, although not diagnostic, can be an objective adjunct to the clinical diagnosis of FTS.[3,50] Again, these markers can be used to trend treatment response.[51] In a study of 71 patients with FTS, elevation of all 3 markers had a specificity and positive predictive value of 100% when correlated with intraoperative findings or cultures. Baseline values used for WBC count, ESR, and CRP levels were defined as 11,000 cells/mL, 15 mm/h, and less than 1.0 mg/dL, respectively. The sensitivity was 39%, 41%, and 76% and the negative predictive value was 4%, 3%, and 13% for WBC count, ESR, and levels, respectively.[50] At least 1 marker was elevated in all cases, resulting in a sensitivity of 100%.[50] These statistics should be interpreted with caution, because these are markers of inflammation and not specific to FTS.[52]

Radiographs should be obtained to evaluate for foreign bodies or fractures but are often of limited use in evaluating soft tissues.[51] US has been reported to be helpful for early detection of FTS, demonstrating thickening of the tendon and tendon sheath.[23] The synovial sheath is usually thickened, hypoechoic, and hyperemic on Doppler

US, differentiating it from synovial sheath effusion[14,23,53] (**Fig. 13**). In 1 study of patients with an uncertain FTS diagnosis, the presence of either synovial sheath effusion greater than the contralateral finger or synovial sheath thickening had a sensitivity of 94.4%, specificity of 74.4%, positive predictive value of 63%, and negative predictive value of 96.7%.[53]

CT and MRI can demonstrate tenosynovitis and involvement of deep spaces, such as radial-ulnar bursae or the space of Parona (**Fig. 14**).[23,54] The synovitis usually enhances on postcontrast images.[54]

NECROTIZING FASCIITIS

Necrotizing fasciitis or necrotizing soft tissue infection (NSTI) is an infection characterized by necrosis of the fascia with relative sparing of the underlying muscle.[3] The disease is potentially fatal and requires immediate clinical, laboratory, and radiographic assessment. Diagnosis is confirmed by frozen section, which will show thrombosis obliterans of the perforating vessels and massive infiltration of polymorphonuclear cells.[18]

Gas in the tissue can be seen on radiographs and is considered a definitive sign of NSTI in the

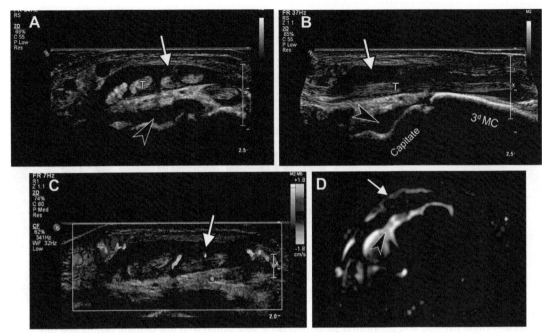

Fig. 13. Tenosynovitis of the fourth extensor compartment in a 62-year-old diabetic man. (*A*) Transverse and (*B*) longitudinal grayscale and (*C*) transverse color Doppler US images of the dorsum of the hand show complex fluid and hyperemia in the tendon sheath (*arrows; A–C*; T, tendon); note midcarpal joint effusion (*arrowhead*). Axial STIR image (*D*) at the same level as (*A*) depicts joint effusion (*arrowhead*) and tenosynovial fluid (*arrow*). Note superior spatial resolution of US in evaluation of superficial soft tissue structures compared with MRI.

appropriate clinical situation.[55–57] Unfortunately, small gas bubbles adjacent to fascial planes have low sensitivity.[33,38,39] X rays are usually unremarkable until the infection and necrosis are advanced.

US has limited use in the actual diagnosis of necrotizing fasciitis but can be used as an adjunct to assist in early diagnosis. Distorted and thickened fascial planes with hypoechoic fluid accumulations in the fascial layers and air present in the soft tissues can be observed.[58]

In challenging cases, advanced imaging is an invaluable adjunct to clinical and laboratory examination. Although most imaging findings lack specificity, CT and MRI help delineate the extent of the disease and provide information for surgical planning.[59] It should be emphasized that absence of soft tissue gas on imaging does not exclude NSTE, because identification of gas has high specificity but low sensitivity.

In addition to delineating the overall disease extent, MRI may demonstrate findings that can help differentiate necrotizing from nonnecrotizing fasciitis, depicting severity and extent of deep fascial involvement and muscle involvement.[23,60] It should be noted that adjacent reactive edema may exaggerate the pathologic condition, whereas

diminished vascular perfusion and tissue necrosis may diminish the degree of contrast enhancement.[57,61] The sensitivity and specificity of MRI in the detection of NSTI have been reported to be 89% to 100% and 46% to 86%, respectively.[59]

CT is a quick and accessible tool for NSTI diagnosis. It is the most sensitive imaging modality for the detection of soft tissue gas.[59,62] The hallmarks of NSTI are edema and asymmetrical thickening of the deep fascial layers. In addition, stranding of the subcutaneous fat, fluid collections along the facial planes, and muscle enhancement can be appreciated.[56,63]

Laboratory evaluation is mandatory but should not delay surgical debridement. Certain laboratory values are independent predictors of death, including WBC count greater than 30,000 and creatinine level greater than 2.[64] The laboratory risk indicator for necrotizing fasciitis (LRINEC) score is used to assist in diagnosis. The score includes CRP level, WBC count, hemoglobin, sodium, creatinine, and glucose levels. A score of 8 or more indicates there is more than a 75% chance of having a necrotizing infection.[65]

Apart from LRINEC, sodium level and WBC count alone are helpful to increase clinical suspicion for NSTI and also aid in diagnosis.[66,67] Wall

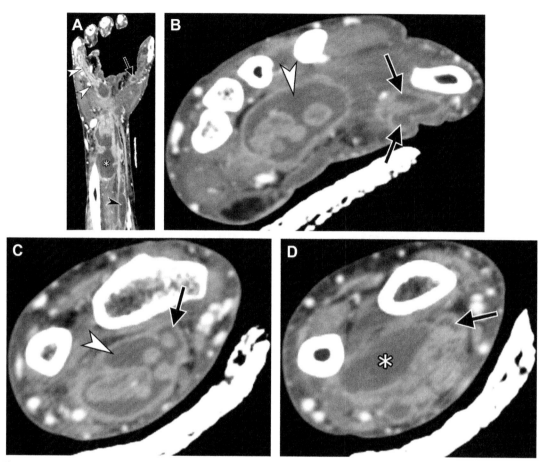

Fig. 14. Pyogenic FTS and deep space infection in a 47-year-old man, chronically immunosuppressed from steroid treatment. (*A*) Contrast-enhanced coronal reformatted and (*B–D*) axial images of the upper extremity demonstrate distended radial (*arrow*) and ulnar (*white arrowheads*) bursae with thick enhancing tenosynovium. (*C*) The bursae communicate at the wrist and connect to a collection in the space of Parona (*asterisk; A, D*). Additional collection is seen in the deep soft tissues of the forearm (*black arrowhead; A*). Short scanning time of CT allows imaging of large anatomic areas when patients cannot tolerate longer MRI scan time.

and colleagues[67] found the combination of a WBC greater than 15,400 cells/mL and serum-sodium level less than 135 mmol/L to have a negative predictive value of 99% and a positive predictive value of 26% for NSTI.

Neeki and colleagues[68] recently brought into question the utility of the LRINEC in differentiating cellulitis and NSTI in the ER setting. In their retrospective series, a high false positive rate was encountered. More than 10% of patients with cellulitis were at moderately high risk for NSTI based on LRINEC score. Furthermore, more than half of the patients with NSTI were low risk based on LRINEC score. The study did find that the LRINEC score performed better in patients with diabetes, with significant differences in WBC count, sodium creatinine, glucose, and CRP levels but not hemoglobin level.[68]

SUMMARY

A spectrum of clinical manifestations of hand infection and complex anatomy of the hand can impede diagnosis. Correlation of clinical findings with laboratory and imaging results greatly enhances the clinician's ability to provide timely diagnosis. Easily accessible and cost-effective imaging techniques like radiography and US should be routinely used during evaluation. The use of CT and MRI should be tailored to specific clinical scenarios. Inflammatory markers should also be evaluated in the appropriate setting to establish diagnosis and also monitor disease progression after treatment. Because hand infections are associated with significant morbidity, it is vital that clinicians use all tools available to make a prompt and accurate diagnosis.

DISCLOSURE

The authors have nothing to disclose.

REFERENCES

1. Mcdonald LS, Bavaro MF, Hofmeister EP, et al. Hand infections. J Hand Surg Am 2011;36(8):1403–12.
2. Franko OI, Abrams RA. Hand infections. Orthop Clin North Am 2013;44(4):625–34.
3. Osterman M, Draeger R, Stern P. Acute hand infections. J Hand Surg Am 2014;39(8):1628–35.
4. Howell JD. Early clinical use of the X-ray. Trans Am Clin Climatol Assoc 2016;127:341–9.
5. Rubin GD. Computed tomography: revolutionizing the practice of medicine for 40 years. Radiology 2014;273(2 Suppl):45–74.
6. Ahlawat S, Corl FM, LaPorte DM, et al. MDCT of hand and wrist infections: emphasis on compartmental anatomy. Clin Radiol 2017;72(4):338.e1-9.
7. Mallinson PI, Coupal TM, Mclaughlin PD, et al. Dual-energy CT for the musculoskeletal system. Radiology 2016;281(3):690–707.
8. Bandettini PA. Twenty years of functional MRI: the science and the stories. Neuroimage 2012;62(2):575–88.
9. Anderson ML, Skinner JA, Felmlee JP, et al. Diagnostic comparison of 1.5 Tesla and 3.0 Tesla preoperative MRI of the wrist in patients with ulnar-sided wrist pain. J Hand Surg Am 2008;33(7):1153–9.
10. Saupe N. 3-Tesla high-resolution MR imaging of the wrist. Semin Musculoskelet Radiol 2009;13(1):29–38.
11. Dewan AK, Chhabra AB, Khanna AJ, et al. Magnetic resonance imaging of the hand and wrist: techniques and spectrum of disease: AAOS exhibit selection. J Bone Joint Surg Am 2013;95(10):e68.
12. Ochman S, Wieskötter B, Langer M, et al. High-resolution MRI (3T-MRI) in diagnosis of wrist pain: is diagnostic arthroscopy still necessary? Arch Orthop Trauma Surg 2017;137(10):1443–50.
13. Gottlieb J, Mailhot T, Chilstrom M. Point-of-care ultrasound diagnosis of deep space hands ultrasound in the diagnosis of complex hand infections: a case series. J Emerg Med 2015;48(1):63–8.
14. Marvel BA, Budhram GR. Bedside ultrasound in the diagnosis of complex hand infections: a case series. J Emerg Med 2015;48(1):63–8.
15. Bray C, Bell LN, Liang H, et al. Erythrocyte sedimentation rate and C-reactive protein measurements and their relevance in clinical medicine. WMJ 2016;115(6):317–21.
16. van Leeuwen MA, van Rijswijk MH. Acute phase proteins in the monitoring of inflammatory disorders. Baillieres Clin Rheumatol 1994;8(3):531–52.
17. Michail M, Jude E, Liaskos C, et al. The performance of serum inflammatory markers for the diagnosis and follow-up of patients with osteomyelitis. Int J Low Extrem Wounds 2013;12(2):94–9.
18. Wolfe SW, Pederson WC, Hotchkiss RN, et al. Green's operative hand surgery: the pediatric hand E-book. Philadelphia: Elsevier Health Sciences; 2010.
19. Berbari E, Mabry T, Tsaras G, et al. Inflammatory blood laboratory levels as markers of prosthetic joint infection. J Bone Joint Surg Am 2010;92(11):2102–9.
20. Simon L, Gauvin F, Amre DK, et al. Serum procalcitonin and C-reactive protein levels as markers of bacterial infection: a systematic review and meta-analysis. Clin Infect Dis 2004;39(2):206–17.
21. Kothari NA, Pelchovitz DJ, Meyer JS. Imaging of musculoskeletal infections. Radiol Clin North Am 2001;39(4):653–71.
22. Loyer EM, DuBrow RA, David CL, et al. Imaging of superficial soft-tissue infections: sonographic findings in cases of cellulitis and abscess. AJR Am J Roentgenol 1996;166(1):149–52.
23. Patel DB, Emmanuel NB, Stevanovic MV, et al. Hand infections: anatomy, types and spread of infection, imaging findings, and treatment options. Radiographics 2014;34(7):1968–86.
24. Chau CL, Griffith JF. Musculoskeletal infections: ultrasound appearances. Clin Radiol 2005;60(2):149–59.
25. Struk DW, Munk PL, Lee MJ, et al. Imaging of soft tissue infections. Radiol Clin North Am 2001;39(2):277–303.
26. Ma LD, Frassica FJ, Bluemke DA, et al. CT and MRI evaluation of musculoskeletal infection. Crit Rev Diagn Imaging 1997;38(6):535–68.
27. Charles HW. Abscess drainage. Semin Intervent Radiol 2012;29(4):325–36.
28. Burkhalter WE. Deep space infections. Hand Clin 1989;5(4):553–9.
29. Chang CD, Wu JS. Imaging of musculoskeletal soft tissue infection. Semin Roentgenol 2017;52(1):55–62.
30. Gaspari R, Dayno M, Briones J, et al. Comparison of computerized tomography and ultrasound for diagnosing soft tissue abscesses. Crit Ultrasound J 2012;4(1):5.
31. Tayal VS, Hasan N, Norton HJ, et al. The effect of soft-tissue ultrasound on the management of cellulitis in the emergency department. Acad Emerg Med 2006;13(4):384–8.
32. Turecki MB, Taljanovic MS, Stubbs AY, et al. Imaging of musculoskeletal soft tissue infections. Skeletal Radiol 2010;39(10):957–71.
33. Stalcup ST, Pathria MN, Hughes TH. Musculoskeletal infections of the extremities: a tour from superficial to deep. Appl Radiol 2011;40(11):12.
34. de Mooij T, Riester S, Kakar S. Key MR imaging features of common hand surgery conditions. Magn Reson Imaging Clin N Am 2015;23(3):495–510.

35. Maharajan K, Patro DK, Menon J, et al. Serum procalcitonin is a sensitive and specific marker in the diagnosis of septic arthritis and acute osteomyelitis. J Orthop Surg Res 2013;4(8):19.

36. Li SF, Cassidy C, Chang C, et al. Diagnostic utility of laboratory tests in septic arthritis. Emerg Med J 2007;24(2):75–7.

37. Lenski M, Scherer MA. Analysis of synovial inflammatory markers to differ infectious from gouty arthritis. Clin Biochem 2014;47(1–2):49–55.

38. Theodorou SJ, Theodorou DJ, Resnick D. Imaging findings of complications affecting the upper extremity in intravenous drug users: featured cases. Emerg Radiol 2008;15(4):227–39.

39. Lalam RK, Cassar-Pullicino VN, Tins BJ. Magnetic resonance imaging of appendicular musculoskeletal infection. Top Magn Reson Imaging 2007;18(3): 177–91.

40. Graif M, Schweitzer ME, Deely D, et al. The septic versus nonseptic inflamed joint: MRI characteristics. Skeletal Radiol 1999;28(11):616–20.

41. Pinder R, Barlow G. Osteomyelitis of the hand. J Hand Surg Eur Vol 2016;41(4):431–40.

42. Mouzopoulos G, Kanakaris NK, Kontakis G, et al. Management of bone infections in adults: the surgeon's and microbiologist's perspectives. Injury 2011;42(Suppl 5):S18–23.

43. Honda H, McDonald JR. Current recommendations in the management of osteomyelitis of the hand and wrist. J Hand Surg Am 2009;34(6):1135–6.

44. Reilly KE, Linz JC, Stern PJ, et al. Osteomyelitis of the tubular bones of the hand. J Hand Surg Am 1997;22(4):644–9.

45. Lin Z, Vasudevan A, Tambyah PA. Use of erythrocyte sedimentation rate and C-reactive protein to predict osteomyelitis recurrence. J Orthop Surg (Hong Kong) 2016;24(1):77–83.

46. Shen CJ, Wu MS, Lin K, et al. The use of procalcitonin in the diagnosis of bone and joint infection: a systemic review and meta-analysis. Eur J Clin Microbiol Infect Dis 2013;32(6):807–14.

47. Klosterhalfen B, Peters KM, Tons C, et al. Local and systemic inflammatory mediator release in patients with acute and chronic posttraumatic osteomyelitis. J Trauma 1996;40(3):372–8.

48. Jungmann PM, Agten CA, Pfirrmann CW, et al. Advances in MRI around metal. J Magn Reson Imaging 2017;46(4):972–91.

49. Brenner AI, Koshy J, Morey J, et al. The bone scan. Semin Nucl Med 2012;42(1):11–26.

50. Bishop GB, Born T, Kakar S, et al. The diagnostic accuracy of inflammatory blood markers for purulent flexor tenosynovitis. J Hand Surg Am 2013;38(11): 2208–11.

51. Draeger RW, Bynum DK Jr. Flexor tendon sheath infections of the hand. J Am Acad Orthop Surg 2012; 20(6):373–82.

52. Hyatt BT, Bagg MR. Flexor tenosynovitis. Orthop Clin North Am 2017;48(2):217–27.

53. Jardin E, Delord M, Aubry S, et al. Usefulness of ultrasound for the diagnosis of pyogenic flexor tenosynovitis: a prospective single-center study of 57 cases. Hand Surg Rehabil 2018;37(2):95–8.

54. Reinus WR, De Cotiis D, Schaffer A. Changing patterns of septic tenosynovitis of the distal extremities. Emerg Radiol 2015;22(2):133–9.

55. Wong CH, Khin LW. Clinical relevance of the LRINEC (Laboratory Risk Indicator for Necrotizing Fasciitis) score for assessment of early necrotizing fasciitis. Crit Care Med 2005;33(7):1677.

56. Fugitt JB, Puckett ML, Quigley MM, et al. Necrotizing fasciitis. Radiographics 2004;24(5):1472–6.

57. Anaya DA, Dellinger EP. Necrotizing soft-tissue infection: diagnosis and management. Clin Infect Dis 2007;44(5):705–10.

58. Chao HC, Kong MS, Lin TY. Diagnosis of necrotizing fasciitis in children. J Ultrasound Med 1999;18(4): 277–81.

59. Paz Maya S, Dualde Beltrán D, Lemercier P, et al. Necrotizing fasciitis: an urgent diagnosis. Skeletal Radiol 2014;43(5):577–89.

60. Kim KT, Kim YJ, Won Lee J, et al. Can necrotizing infectious fasciitis be differentiated from nonnecrotizing infectious fasciitis with MR imaging? Radiology 2011;259(3):816–24.

61. Schmid MR, Kossmann T, Duewell S. Differentiation of necrotizing fasciitis and cellulitis using MR imaging. AJR Am J Roentgenol 1998;170(3):615–20.

62. Wysoki MG, Santora TA, Shah RM, et al. Necrotizing fasciitis: CT characteristics. Radiology 1997;203(3): 859–63.

63. Berger T, Garrido F, Green J, et al. Bedside ultrasound performed by novices for the detection of abscess in ED patients with soft tissue infections. Am J Emerg Med 2012;30(8):1569–73.

64. Koshy JC, Bell B. Hand infections. J Hand Surg Am 2019;44(1):46–54.

65. Wong CH, Wang YS. The diagnosis of necrotizing fasciitis. Curr Opin Infect Dis 2005;18(2):101–6.

66. Chan T, Yaghoubian A, Rosing D, et al. Low sensitivity of physical examination findings in necrotizing soft tissue infection is improved with laboratory values: a prospective study. Am J Surg 2008; 196(6):926–30.

67. Wall DB, Klein SR, Black S, et al. A simple model to help distinguish necrotizing fasciitis from nonnecrotizing soft tissue infection. J Am Coll Surg 2000; 191(3):227–31.

68. Neeki MM, Dong F, Au C, et al. Evaluating the laboratory risk indicator to differentiate cellulitis from necrotizing fasciitis in the emergency department. West J Emerg Med 2017;18(4):684–9.

Antibiotic Management and Antibiotic Resistance in Hand Infections

Jessica M. Intravia, MD*, Meredith N. Osterman, MD, Rick Tosti, MD

KEYWORDS

- Antibiotic resistance • Community-acquired methicillin-resistant *Staphylococcus aureus*
- Health care–associated methicillin-resistant *Staphylococcus aureus*

KEY POINTS

- Since 1961, the prevalence of methicillin-resistant *Staphylococcus aureus* (MRSA) hand infections has been increasing in both pediatric and adult populations.
- Many hospitals report a greater than 50% prevalence of MRSA in the adult population.
- The mechanism of resistance to methicillin involves the mecA gene, which codes for a mutant penicillin-binding protein 2A.
- For patients with minimal comorbidities in whom outpatient therapy is appropriate, trimethoprim-sulfamethoxazole or doxycycline can be a good choice to cover for MRSA.
- For patients with comorbidities or severe illnesses with systemic signs that require intravenous antibiotics, intravenous vancomycin often is the drug of choice.

INTRODUCTION

Historically, *Staphylococcus aureus* and β-hemolytic streptococci are the most commonly cultured organisms in hand infections. Houshian and colleagues[1] described *Staphylococcus aureus* as the sole cause of hand infections in 44% of 418 patients in their series. Likewise, Stevenson and Anderson[2] found *Staphylococcus aureus* as the source of 42% of hand infections in their series of 160 patients. Alternatively Dellinger and colleagues[3] reported a mixed culture of both *Staphylococcus* and *Streptococcus* species as being most common, because it was present in 84% of patients. Stern and colleagues[4] echoed these results, reporting a mixed culture in 63% of patients.

Methicillin resistance to *Staphylococcus aureus* was first described in the early 1960s, shortly after the introduction of methicillin. Methicillin first was introduced to treat penicillin G–resistant staphylococcus in 1959.[5] Unfortunately, by 1961, *S aureus* bacteria had been isolated that exhibited resistance to methicillin. In 1968, the first large

outbreak of MRSA was reported at Boston City Hospital.[6] Over the following 3 decades, additional cases of resistance were reported. Typically these cases were hospital acquired or confined to the hospital setting.[7] In 1981, however, the first report of a new strain of community-acquired (CA)-MRSA emerged.[8] By the mid-1990s, the acquisition of MRSA in younger and otherwise healthy individuals was alarmingly high, thus beginning the concept of CA-MRSA infections.[9,10] People who worked or lived in close quarters, including prisons, day care centers, schools, and athletic or military settings, were particularly at risk.

PREVALENCE OF METHICILLIN-RESISTANT *STAPHYLOCOCCUS AUREUS*

Since the initial published case reports describing MRSA infections of the hand, the prevalence has been rising.[11–14] One meta-analysis indicated that the prevalence of CA-MRSA in all soft tissue infections was 30% in 27 retrospective studies and 37% in 5 prospective studies from 1983 to 2001.[15]

Philadelphia Hand to Shoulder Center, 834 Chestnut Street, Philadelphia, PA 19107, USA
* Corresponding author.
E-mail address: jintravia@gmail.com

Hand Clin 36 (2020) 301–305
https://doi.org/10.1016/j.hcl.2020.03.003
0749-0712/20/© 2020 Published by Elsevier Inc.

An 8-year longitudinal study at an urban hospital from 2005 to 2012 found methicillin-resistant *Staphylococcus aureus* (MRSA) in 49% of 683 culture positive hand infections, with the annual incidence peaking at 65% in 2007. Over this same time period, concomitant clindamycin resistance in MRSA significantly increased, approaching 20% by 2012. Concomitant levofloxacin resistance also increased to 50%. Sporadic resistance to trimethoprim-sulfamethoxazole (TMP-SMX), tetracycline, gentamicin, and moxifloxacin also was observed. In this study, no resistance was observed to vancomycin, daptomycin, linezolid, and rifampin.[16]

Imahara and Friedrich[17] performed a retrospective review of 159 hand infections treated surgically over an 11-year period from 1997 to 2007. During this study period, the risk of having a CA-MRSA infection was 41% higher with each progressive calendar year relative to the incidence of non-MRSA infections. Intravenous (IV) drug use was an independent risk factor for operatively treated CA-MRSA infections. Similarly, a study out of Parkland Hospital in Dallas, Texas, showed that the percent of CA-MRSA hand infections almost doubled from 2001 to 2003. In their institution, the rate of CA-MRSA infections was 34% in 2001% and 61% in 2003.[18] A 2007 study from Cook County Hospital in Chicago, Illinois, showed MRSA positive cultures in an alarming 73.1% of hand infections treated over a 9-month period.[19]

CA-MRSA infections also are a concern in the pediatric population. A 2012 study, performed in a pediatric emergency room, noted that the prevalence of CA-MRSA in all anatomic sites had doubled between 2003 and 2008. CA-MRSA was found responsible for up to 42% of culture-positive infections.[20] A second study examined skin and soft tissue infections in the hand and demonstrated a 30% prevalence of CA-MRSA infections in healthy patients younger than 15 years of age.[21] Although the prevalence of CA-MRSA in the pediatric population appears lower than that of the adult population, it still raises concern in the treatment of pediatric patients particularly in urban areas.

MECHANISM OF METHICILLIN RESISTANCE

The mechanism of penicillin resistance features β-lactamases and is different from the mechanism of methicillin resistance, which features the mecA gene. In penicillin resistance, β-lactamases secreted by the staphylococcal species hydrolyze the β-lactam ring that forms the foundation of the penicillin. Because methicillin is a semisynthetic penicillin, it is not affected by β-lactamase.

Methicillin resistance is conferred on the presence of the mecA gene, which encodes for a mutant penicillin-binding protein 2A.[22] In general, penicillins and methicillin work by attaching to a protein in the bacterial cell wall called penicillin-binding protein 2, which inhibits the cross-linking of the cell wall. This results in a weakened cell wall and facilitates destruction of the bacteria. In MRSA, the mecA gene codes for a mutant penicillin-binding protein 2A. This mutant protein does not allow penicillins and cephalosporin to bind to the cell wall.[5]

The mecA gene is located on the staphylococcal cassette chromosome mec (*SSCmec*) and is highly transmissible by plasmid transfer. Distinct from the health care–associated type, community-acquired MRSA has a smaller, more mobile cassette.[7] Furthermore, pulsed-field gel electrophoresis patterns of bacterial DNA have identified the CA-MRSA to be mainly USA300 and USA400 strains. CA-MRSA also frequently carries the Panton-Valentine leukocidin (*PVL*) gene, which is seen less commonly in the health care–associated form.[22] The Panton-Valentine leukocidin is a protein that is toxic to host phagocytes. It forms pores in leukocytes, thus facilitating their destruction.

MULTIDRUG-RESISTANT *STAPHYLOCOCCUS AUREUS*

As MRSA becomes increasingly common in both the community and hospital settings, multiple antibiotics are being prescribed to treat these infections. This raises concern for multidrug-resistant staphylococcus species. Tosti and colleagues[23] found that younger age, IV drug use, and nosocomial acquired MRSA were significant risk factors for concurrent clindamycin resistance. Patients with a history of IV drug abuse were 11-times more likely to have concurrent clindamycin resistance. In the event of clindamycin sensitivity with erythromycin resistance, a double-disk diffusion test should be obtained to examine the possibility of erythromycin-induced clindamycin resistance, which can lead to treatment failure.

TREATMENT

The primary treatment of a suspected abscess, felon, paronychia, or flexor tenosynovitis is operative irrigation and débridement. For simple abscesses, thorough incision and drainage often are adequate. If the infection is inadequately débrided, severe with rapid progression, or associated with systemic illness, elderly patients, comorbidities, or immunosuppression, however, then the Infectious Diseases Society of America recommends continued antibiotic therapy.[24]

Empiric antibiotic treatment should target the most likely pathogen until culture sensitivities have been obtained. **Table 1** provides some antibiotic recommendations for commonly encountered organisms.

The Centers for Disease Control and Prevention recommend empiric coverage for MRSA if the local prevalence exceeds 10% to 15%.[25] **Table 2** highlights some antibiotic options used to treat MRSA. Unless the local prevalence of MRSA is limited, first-generation cephalosporins should be avoided as first-line empiric treatment of hand infections. For patients with minimal comorbidities in whom outpatient therapy is appropriate, TMP-SMX can be a good choice to cover for MRSA.

Table 1
Antibiotic recommendations for common organisms

Organism	Antibiotic	Additional Information
Methicillin-sensitive *Staphylococcus aureus*	Cephalexin amoxicillin clavulanate (orally)	
MRSA	TMP-SMX (orally) Linezolid (orally or IV) If sulfa allergy, clindamycin or doxycycline Vancomycin (IV) Daptomycin (IV) Quinupristin/dalfopristin (IV) Tigecycline (IV) Cetaroline (IV)	Linezolid: expensive, avoid in endocarditis or meningitis, weekly complete blood cell monitoring Daptomycin: weekly creatinine phosphokinase monitoring
Vancomycin-resistant enterococci	Daptomycin Linezolid (orally or IV) Tigecycline (IV) Quinupristin/dalfopristin (IV)	
Gram negative	Piperacillin/tazobactam Ceftriaxone Ertapenem Quinolones/ciprofloxacin	
Pseudomonas	Piperacillin/tazobactam Cefepime Meropenem	
Anaerobic infections	Ampicillin/sulbactam, piperacillin/tazobactam Ertapenem Meropenem Metronidazole Clindamycin Tigecycline	
Vibrio vulnificus	Ceftriaxone and doxycycline Imipenem and doxycycline	
Nocardia	TMP-SMX If sulfa allergy: imipenem, ceftriaxone, amikacin	6 mo of treatment in immunosuppressed patients
Sporothrix schenckii	Itraconazole Fluconazole and voriconazole	
Mycobacterium marinum	Clarithromycin/azithromycin TMP-SMX minocycline Ethambutol	
Aeromonas hydrophilia	Ciprofloxacin Imipenem TMP-SMX	
Cutaneous anthrax	Ciprofloxacin Doxycycline	Treatment for 60 d to treat any remaining spores
Tularemia	Gentamicin and doxycycline	

From Osterman M, Draeger R, Stern P. Acute Hand Infections. J Hand Surg Am 2014;39(8):1630; with permission.

Table 2
Summary of antibiotics used to treat methicillin-resistant _Staphylococcus aureus_

Antibiotic	Route of Administration	Benefits	Side Effects
Erythromycin	orally/IV	Good activity against gram-positive organisms	Gastrointestinal side effects, frequent administration
Clindamycin	orally/IV	Good bone penetration	Risk of _Clostridium difficile_ diarrhea
Linezolid	orally/IV	Good bioavailability, low resistance	Hematologic side effects
Daptomycin	IV	Once-daily administration	
Vancomycin	IV	Good experience with use	Nephrotoxicity requires monitoring
Teicoplanin	IV	Less nephrotoxic than vancomycin, daily administration	
Doxycycline	orally	Once-daily administration	Gastrointestinal side effects
Tigecycline	IV	Covers some gram-negative organisms	Gastrointestinal side effects
Rifampin	orally/IV	Good tissue penetration	Cannot be used alone
TMP-SMX	orally	Twice daily oral administration	Gastrointestinal side effects, Stevens-Johnson syndrome

From Harrison B, Ben-Amotz O, Sammer DM. Methicillin-Resistant Staphylococcus aureus Infection in the Hand. Plast Reconstr Surg 2015;135(3):826-830; with permission.

Clindamycin is another alternative. One benefit of clindamycin is its excellent oral bioavailability. The oral bioavailability of clindamycin is approximately 90% of that of the parenteral form. Regional clindamycin resistance, however, also is on the rise. Tetracyclines are another option, especially in those with a sulfa allergy. One study showed an 83% cure rate in CA-MRSA soft tissue infections using doxycycline and minocycline.[26] Rifampin occasionally is used but only in combination with doxycycline or TMP-SMX because high mutation rates can induce resistance. Fluoroquinolones should not be used because resistance develops quickly.[7]

Patients with comorbidities or severe illnesses with systemic signs often require IV antibiotics. IV vancomycin often is the drug of choice. Unfortunately, it has poor oral bioavailability and resistance has been reported.[27] Other IV options include clindamycin, linezolid, tigecycline, daptomycin, quinupristin, and dalfopristin.[7]

SUMMARY

Since 1961, the rates of both CA-MRSA and health care–associated MRSA hand infections have increased rapidly. Treating physicians should be concerned about potential MRSA infections and choose empiric antibiotics to cover MRSA if the local prevalence exceeds 10% to 15%. The authors recommend TMP-SMX or doxycycline for patients with minimal comorbidities in whom outpatient therapy is appropriate. For patients with comorbidities or severe illnesses with systemic signs that require IV antibiotics, IV vancomycin often is the drug of choice.

DISCLOSURE

The authors have nothing to disclose.

REFERENCES

1. Houshian S, Seyedipour S, Weddwerkopp N. Epidemiology of bacterial hand infections. Int J Infect Dis 2006;10(4):315–9.
2. Stevenson J, Anderson IWR. Hand infections: an audit of 160 infections treated in an accident and emergency department. J Hand Surg 1993;18B: 115–8.
3. Dellinger EP, Wertz MJ, Miller SD, et al. Hand infections. Arch Surg 1988;123:745–50.
4. Stern PJ, Staneck JL, McDonough JJ, et al. Established hand infections: a controlled prospective study. J Hand Surg 1983;8:553–9.
5. Harrison B, Ben-Amotz O, Sammer D. Methicillin-resistant _Staphylococcus aureus_ infection in the hand. Plast Reconstr Surg 2015;135:826–30.
6. Barrett FF, McGehee RF Jr, Finland M. Methicillin-resistant _Staphylococcus aureus_ at Boston City

Hospital: Bacteriologic and epidemiologic observations. N Engl J Med 1968;279:441–8.

7. Daum RS. Clinical practice. Skin and soft-tissue infections caused by methicillin-resistant Staphylococcus aureus. N Engl J Med 2007;357:380–90.

8. Pottinger PS. Methicillin-resistant *Staphlococcus aureus* infections. Med Clin North Am 2013;97: 601–19.

9. Herold BC, Immergluck LC, Maranan MC, et al. Community-acquired methicillin-resistant Staphylococcus aureus in children with no predisposing risk. JAMA 1998;279:593–8.

10. From the Centers for Disease Control and Prevention. Four pediatric deaths from community-acquired methicillin-resistant Staphylococcus aureus–Minnesota and North Dakota, 1997–1999. JAMA 1999;282:1123–5.

11. Karanas YL, Bogdan MA, Chang J. Community acquired methicillin-resistant Staphylococcus aureus hand infections: case reports and clinical implications. J Hand Surg 2000;25A:760–3.

12. Connolly B, Johnstone F, Gerlinger T, et al. Methicillin-resistant Staphylococcus aureus in a finger felon. J Hand Surg Am 2000;25A:173–5.

13. Berlet G, Richards RS, Roth JH. Clenched fist injury complicated by MRSA. Can J Surg 1997;40:313–4.

14. Gelfand MS. Hand infection and bacteremia due to methicillin-resistant Staphylococcus aureus following a clenched-fist injury in a nursing home resident. Clin Infect Dis 1994;18:469.

15. Salgado CD, Farr BM, Calfee DP. Community-acquired methicillin- resistant Staphylococcus aureus: a meta-analysis of prevalence and risk factors. Clin Infect Dis 2003;36:131–9.

16. Tosti R, Samuelsen BT, Bender S, et al. Emerging multidrug resistance of methicillin-resistant Staphylococcus aureus in hand infections. J Bone Joint Surg Am 2014;96(18):1535–40.

17. Imahara SD, Friedrich JB. Community-acquired methicillin-resistant *Staphylococcus aureus* in surgically treated hand infections. J Hand Surg 2010; 35A:97–103.

18. LeBlanc DM, Reece EM, Horton JB, et al. Increasing incidence of methicillin-resistant *Staphylococcus*
aureus in hand infections: a 3-year county hospital experience. Plast Reconstr Surg 2007;119:935–40.

19. Bach HG, Steffin B, Chhadia AM, et al. Community-associated methicillin-resistant *Staphylococcus aureus* hand infections in an urban setting. J Hand Surg 2007;32A:380–3.

20. Karamatsu ML, Thorp AW, Brown L. Changes in community-associated methicillin-resistant *Staphylococcus aureus* skin and soft tissue infections presenting to the pediatric emergency department: Comparing 2003-2008. Pediatr Emerg Care 2012; 28:131–5.

21. Chung MT, Wilcon P, Rinker B. Community-acquired methicillin resistant *Staphylococcus aureus* hand infections in the pediatric population. J Hand Surg Am 2012;37:326–31.

22. Bassetti M, Nicco E, Mikulska M. Why is community-associated MRSA spreading across the world and how will it change clinical practice? Int J Antimicrob Agents 2009;34(Suppl 1):S15–9.

23. Tosti R, Trionfo A, Gaughan J, et al. Risk factors associated with clindamycin-resistant, methicillin-resistant *Staphylococcus aureus* in hand abscesses. J Hand Surg Am 2015;40(4):673–6.

24. Liu C, Bayer A, Cosgrove SE, et al, Infectious Disease Society of America. Clinical practice guidelines by the infectious diseases society of America for the treatment of methicillin-resistant *Staphylococcus aureus* infections in adults and children. Clin Infect Dis 2011;52:18–55.

25. Gorwitz RJ, Jernigan DB, Powers JH, et al. Participants in the CDC–Convened Experts' Meeting on Management of MRSA in the Community. Strategies for clinical management of MRSA in the com- munity: summary of an experts' meeting convened by the CDC. Atlanta (GA): Centers for Disease Control and Prevention; 2006.

26. Ruhe JJ, Monson T, Bradsher RW, et al. Use of long-acting tetracyclines for methicillin-resistant Staphylococcus aureus infections: case series and review of the literature. Clin Infect Dis 2005;40:1429–34.

27. Smith TL, Pearson ML, Wilcox KR, et al. Emergence of vancomycin resistance in Staphylococcus aureus. Glycopeptide-intermediate Staphylococcus aureus Working Group. N Engl J Med 1999;340:493–501.

Hand Abscesses
Volar and Dorsal

Mark S. Rekant, MD[a,b,c],*, Ryan Tarr, DO[d]

KEYWORDS

• Hand abscess • Hand infections • Collar button abscess

KEY POINTS

- A high index of suspicion coupled with an excellent knowledge of hand anatomy and function allows for an accurate diagnosis and effective management of deep space infections.
- Drainage, debridement, and intraoperative irrigation are the initial steps along with the decision for continuous postoperative irrigation based on intraoperative findings. In addition, focused and thorough postoperative evaluation and antibiotics are keys to successful management of these soft tissue deep abscesses.
- The wound is closed later or by secondary intention if continuous postoperative irrigation is not used.
- Lastly, it is helpful to involve an experienced hand therapist early in the recovery process to guide wound care along with passive assisted and active range of motion exercises of the wrist and digits.

Common hand infections are divided into superficial and deep with regard to the fascial planes and compartments of the hand. It was not until the mid-1900s, under the study of Dr Allen Kanavel, that the compartments within the hand were well understood. Today, deep-space infections comprise 5% to 15% of all hand infections.[1]

In deep space hand infections, apart of antibiotic coverage and immobilization with hand elevation, the surgical incision and drainage of all potentially communicating spaces and compartments is mandatory. Management should include intraoperative irrigation and sometimes, continuous postoperative irrigation via an indwelling catheter. Such parameters as the pathway of inoculation, the environment where the initial injury occurred, and the underlying condition of the patient need to be taken into consideration for successful treatment. Finally, postoperative hand therapy should be initiated as soon as the acute signs of infections subside.

Antibiotics are usually required for 7 to 10 days unless complications arise.[2] The route of administration is intravenous for all cases that require hospitalization, until the remission of the acute signs of infection. Subsequently an oral regimen could be administered.

Antibiotic treatment is usually initiated with penicillinase-resistant penicillin or cephalosporins. The oral empiric antibiotic treatment expected to be effective against suspected community-acquired methicillin-resistant *Staphylococcus aureus* infections includes ciprofloxacin, clindamycin, rifampin, tetracyclines, and trimethoprim/sulfamethoxazole. For more serious infections, intravenous vancomycin is recommended.

Specific approaches are presented for the different types of closed-space infections. In all cases a bloodless field is imperative for the evaluation of all potentially infected closed-spaces and

---

[a] Philadelphia Hand to Shoulder Center, Philadelphia, PA 19107, USA; [b] Department of Orthopaedic Surgery, Thomas Jefferson University, Philadelphia, PA 19107, USA; [c] Patricia Lincke, 1888 Marlton Pike East, Suite E, Cherry Hill, NJ 08057, USA; [d] Philadelphia Hand to Shoulder Center, The Franklin, Suite G114, 834 Chestnut Street, Philadelphia, PA 19107, USA
* Patricia Lincke, 1888 Marlton Pike East, Suite E, Cherry Hill, NJ 08057.
E-mail address: msrekant@handcenters.com
Twitter: @mrekant (M.S.R.)

Hand Clin 36 (2020) 307–312
https://doi.org/10.1016/j.hcl.2020.03.014
0749-0712/20/© 2020 Elsevier Inc. All rights reserved.

for the drainage through safe anatomic paths. Special attention must be given to the avoidance of use of Esmarch bandage to limit the spread of infection. Simple elevation of the hand and forearm is usually adequate for a proper visualization after inflating the tourniquet.

Deep hand abscesses remain challenging to manage, causing patients significant pain and loss of function. The accumulation of purulent material in this part of the hand raises the pressure within the closed-space, which can lead to ischemia and necrosis of the surrounding soft tissues. Optimal care requires the surgeon to fully understand the anatomy of the hand so that these closed-space abscesses are recognized and treated appropriately. Management usually necessitates adequate incision and drainage, appropriate antibiotic therapy, elevation and edema control, and mobilization. These infections are usually attributed to gram-positive cocci and clinicians should also consider the local spread of community-acquired methicillin-resistant S aureus and the host's comorbidities, such as immunosuppression and diabetes, before choosing the appropriate antibiotics. Staphylococcus is the principal organism in 50% to 80% of infections.[1]

The familiarity of anatomy of the hand, closed-space pathophysiology, and current updates in microbiology and drainage/irrigation techniques are prerequisites for prompt diagnosis and optimal treatment of acute closed-space hand infections. Knowledge of the likely pathogens is based on the history, nature, and course of infection and can direct culture and staining requests. Routine aerobic and anaerobic cultures and Gram stain should be done.

Initial diagnosis may be perplexing; because of the deep location of closed-space accumulations, the typical signs of infection are often absent. A strong index of suspicion is imperative with a patient presenting with throbbing pain, edema, and restricted finger motion because these findings are most common. The physical examination should include a thorough examination of the hand, with particular attention to the following: cellulitis, lymphangitis, areas of fluctuance, and range of motion.

Plain radiographs with a minimum of three views of the hand (anteroposterior, lateral, and oblique) are important for identification of potential presence of foreign bodies, fractures, and subcutaneous air. Subcutaneous air presence typically suggests gas gangrene, whereas radiolucencies are suggestive of acute or chronic osteomyelitis. MRI may be obtained for further evaluation and delineation of soft tissue abscess.

The deep spaces of the hand include the thenar, midpalmar, dorsal subaponeurotic, Parona quadrilateral, and interdigital subfascial web spaces (Fig. 1). These spaces can fill with bacteria and

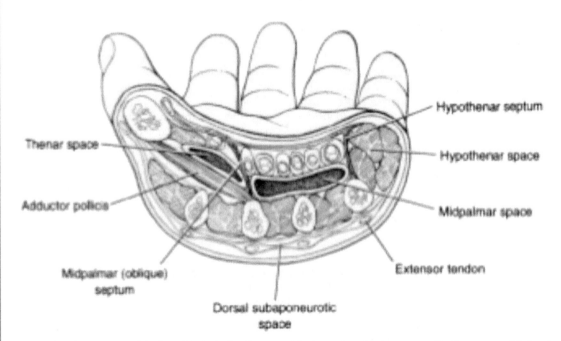

Fig. 1. The deep spaces of the hand include the thenar, midpalmar, dorsal subaponeurotic, Parona quadrilateral, and interdigital subfascial web spaces. (*From* Jamil W, Khan I, Robinson P, et al. Acute compartment syndrome of the forearm secondary to infection within the space of Parona. Orthopedics 2011;34(9):e584-7; with permission.)

purulent material manifesting into abscesses of the thenar space and compartment, the hypothenar space, compartment and the subaponeurotic space of the dorsum of the hand, and the midpalmar space. Deep-space infections usually occur via penetrating inoculation or contiguous spread or extension from adjacent tendon synovium/bursae or fascial spaces; occasionally, hematogenous seeding is responsible. *Streptococcus, S aureus*, and coliform organisms are the most common infectious agents.[1]

The differences between the palmar and dorsal structures may explain the different pathways of extension and the different clinical signs of infection between the two sides of the hand. The palmar skin is thicker than the dorsal and is anchored to the underlying structures. It contains many sweat glands but no hair follicles or sebaceous glands, whereas the tough palmar fascia represents a thick and resistant fibrous tissue layer. Both skin and fascia hinder the horizontal spread of pus and even edema to the palm. Pus is rather oriented to the deeper palmar structures, whereas edema is always more prominent at the dorsum of the hand.[3]

When dealing with thenar compartment and thenar space infections, understanding of the anatomy is paramount. The thenar space is bordered dorsally by the adductor pollicis, palmarly by the index finger flexor tendon, and ulnarly by the midpalmar septum (which extends from the middle finger). On presentation, a painful swelling of the thenar eminence is observed along with tenderness in the palm. The normal concavity of the palm is lost, so that it instead appears flattened or convex. Often, this is accompanied by soft edema on the dorsum of the hand. The thumb metacarpal and the thumb are abducted, and distal phalanx flexion becomes more marked. In extensive infections, a double incision over the volar and dorsal side is necessary for drainage of the infected spaces/compartments (**Fig. 2**).[4–8]

Abscesses within the hypothenar compartment and space infections tend to be more localized. This space contains the hypothenar muscles contained within the muscle fascia. The hypothenar space is unique in that it does not contain any flexor tendons. There is often limited swelling in the palm but always painful swelling of the hypothenar eminence. The incision should be made over the hypothenar region with great caution to avoid injury to the neurovascular bundle.[5]

In a midpalmar infection, the concavity of the palm is also usually absent. The deep palmar space is bordered dorsally by the middle and ring finger metacarpals and the second and third

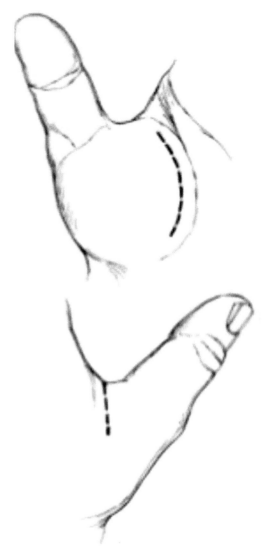

Fig. 2. The volar and dorsal incisions for a thenar abscess. One or both incisions are used for drainage of the infected spaces/compartments. (*From* Seiler JG. Essentials of Hand Surgery. Philadelphia: Lippincott Williams & Wilkins, 2001. Copyright American Society for Surgery of the Hand; with permission.)

palmar interosseous muscles, palmarly by the flexor tendons and lumbricals, radially by the midpalmar septum, and ulnarly by the hypothenar muscles. Direct penetration or, in rare cases, contiguous spread from the flexor sheaths of the middle and ring fingers may cause infection.[9,10] Dorsal hand swelling may be so impressive that the palmar process is overlooked. Passive motion of the middle and ring fingers elicits pain. The fingers are held rigidly flexed, with decreasing rigidity from the fifth digit to the index finger. However, finger rigidity in case of midpalmar infections is less severe than the rigidity of septic tenosynovitis.

Transverse and oblique longitudinal incisions have been described for drainage, and a distal approach in the third interspace, which allows evacuation of the abscess through the lumbrical canal (**Fig. 3**).[11]

Wide exposure and drainage are preferred, after which the wound is either left open and dressed in loose wet-gauze packing (which should be changed daily) or closed over irrigation catheters. Care should be taken to avoid injury of the neurovascular bundles.[6,7,12]

The dorsal subaponeurotic space is contained by the extensor tendons and fascia dorsally and the metacarpals and interosseous muscles palmarly. Infection of this space is accompanied by considerable dorsal hand swelling and may be difficult to distinguish from a subcutaneous abscess. A preferred method of incision and drainage is with two longitudinal incisions (over the second metacarpal and over the interspace between the fourth and fifth metacarpals), followed by local wound care and early motion.[13]

Incisions directly over the digital extensor tendons should be avoided, to prevent compromise of their coverage.

WEB SPACE INFECTIONS

These are either primary infections from direct inoculation or secondary extending from the adjacent anatomic structures. The diagnosis is clinical and based on an abscess forming at the distal edge of the palm separating the adjacent fingers. One such example is a collar button abscess. Closed-space hand infections, such as a collar button abscess, should be drained with urgency. Delay in treatment could result in the spread of infection throughout the deep spaces, risking significant compromise of hand function. Damage to neurovascular structures is possible with incision and drainage, and care should be taken when draining a collar button abscess because of the proximity of the bifurcating common digital nerves and arteries.

The choice of surgical technique is of great importance when treating a collar button abscess.

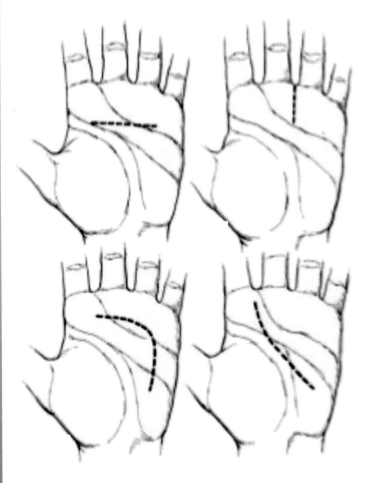

Fig. 3. The volar and dorsal incisions for a thenar abscess. One or both incisions are used for drainage of the infected spaces/compartments. (*From* Seiler JG. Essentials of Hand Surgery. Philadelphia: Lippincott Williams & Wilkins, 2001. Copyright American Society for Surgery of the Hand; with permission.)

Old-fashioned collar buttons were dumbbell shaped; the collar closure was secured by passing the ends of the collar button through overlap ping buttonholes. "Collar-button abscess" describes a subfascial infection of a web space that tends to spread peripherally at the palmar and dorsal ends and remains narrow in the middle. Proper decompression of a collar button abscess always requires volar and dorsal incisions because of the communicating channel between the volar and dorsal hand, which creates an hourglass-shaped abscess.[1] Many incision patterns exist, but treatment should involve two incisions, a longitudinal incision between digits on the dorsal hand and a volar Z-pattern incision.[8] These incisions should extend between the proximal edge of the web and distal palmar crease to avoid the common digital neurovascular bundle. It is important to avoid a transverse web space incision because of the risk of scar contracture leading to a loss of digital abduction.[1,14] Regardless of the incision type, blunt dissection should be used to create a connection between the dorsal and volar extensions of the abscess to avoid damaging the surrounding neurovascular bundles. After the collection of cultures and extensive irrigation, the incisions are left open with the assistance of moist packing or a Penrose drain.[1,8] Drains are typically removed after 24 to 48 hours and followed by hand soaks. Antibiotic therapy serves as an adjunct to surgical intervention.[3] Web space incision should never span transversely across the web space because of scar contracture and subsequent loss of finger abduction.[8]

Collar button abscesses usually result from contiguous spread, most often from an infected palmar blister or skin fissure. Because of the adherence of the palmar skin and underlying fascia, the infection cannot spread peripherally; rather, it is forced to expand dorsally through the space in the palmar fascia (just distal to the bifurcation of the neurovascular bundle) to involve the subcutaneous tissue of the dorsal web.[1,13] Collar button abscesses can also occur from direct inoculation or secondary infection from adjacent anatomic structures.[1–3] S aureus and group A Streptococcus are the most common infectious agents, with S aureus reported to be 30% to 80% of positive cultures.[4]

Similarly, surgical drainage of multiloculated abscesses in the hand incorporating a palmar and a dorsal incision also should never cross the edge of the web to avoid the formation of dysfunctional scars.

Another deep space abscess can include Parona space. The compromise of Parona space usually results from contiguous spread from the radial or ulnar bursa.[15] Symptoms may include acute carpal tunnel syndrome and pain with finger-flexor motion actively and passively. Management is similar to that of other deep-space infections, emphasizing wide exposure and thorough drainage, and avoiding placement of incisions directly over the flexor tendons and the median nerve to avoid desiccation.

If the hand infection has been treated appropriately with measures, such as eradication of the abscess and devitalized tissue, the risk of recurrence is minimal.

In the operating room, perform all explorations and debridements under tourniquet control. The extremity should be exsanguinated by gravity. Obtain wound cultures before the administration of antibiotics; then administer a dose of perioperative antibiotics because of the likelihood of a transient bacteremia after debridement.

The incision should be centered over the area of fluctuance. Incisions are made along the palmar creases when possible. In the case of deep-space infections, wide exposure is important. The palmar fascia is incised, and the common digital nerves and vessels should be identified and protected when possible. A palmar and dorsal incision may be necessary, particularly in the case of collar button abscesses.

Specific approaches have been described for the different types of closed-space infections that will likely been seen throughout a hand surgeon's career. In all cases, a bloodless field is imperative for the evaluation of all potentially infected closed-spaces and for the drainage through safe anatomic pathways. Special attention must be given to the avoidance of use of Esmarch bandage to limit the spread of infection. Simple elevation of the hand and forearm before elevating the tourniquet is usually adequate for a bloodless field.

Drainage, debridement, and intraoperative irrigation are the initial steps, whereas the decision for continuous postoperative irrigation is based on intraoperative findings. Focused and thorough postoperative evaluation and antibiotics are keys to successful management of these soft tissue deep abscesses. The wound can be closed later or by secondary intention if continuous postoperative irrigation is not used.[4,16] Lastly, it is helpful to involve an experienced hand therapist early in the recovery process to guide wound care along with passive assisted and active range of motion exercises of the wrist and digits.

DISCLOSURE

The authors have nothing to disclose.

REFERENCES

1. Hausman MR, Lisser SP. Hand infections. Orthop Clin North Am 1992;23:171–85.
2. Dellinger EP, Wertz MJ, Miller SD, et al. Hand infections. Bacteriology and treatment: a prospective study. Arch Surg 1988;123:745–9.
3. Spann M, Talmor M, Nolan W. Hand infections: basic principles and management. Surg Infect (Larchmt) 2004;5:210–20.
4. Abrams RA, Botte MJ. Hand infections: treatment recommendations for specific types. J Am Acad Orthop Surg 1996;4:219–30.
5. Brown MB, Young LV. Hand infections. South Med J 1993;86:56–66.
6. Shamblin WR. The diagnosis and treatment of acute infections of the hand. South Med J 1969;62:209–12.
7. Robins RHC. Infections of the hand. J Bone Joint Surg Br 1952;34:567–80.
8. Jebson PL. Deep subfascial space infections. Hand Clin 1998;14:557–66.
9. Weinweig N, Gonzalez M. Surgical infections of the hand and upper extremity: a county hospital experience. Ann Plast Surg 2002;49:621–7.
10. Dailiana ZH, Rigopoulos N, Varitimidis S, et al. Purulent flexor tenosynovitis: factors influencing the functional outcome. J Hand Surg Eur 2008;33:280–5.
11. Neviaser RJ. Infections. In: Green DP, editor. Operative hand surgery, vol. 1, 3rd edition. New York: Churchill Livingstone; 1993. p. 1021–38.
12. Kanavel AB. Infections of the hand. 4th edition. Philadelphia: Lea, Febiger; 1921. p. 16.
13. Burkhalter WE. Deep space infections. Hand Clin 1989;5:553–9.
14. Mann RJ, Hoffeld TA, Farmer CB. Human bites of the hand: twenty years of experience. J Hand Surg Am 1977;2:97–104.
15. Best R. An anatomical and clinical study of infections of the hand. Ann Surg 1929;89:359–78.
16. Stomberg BV. Retreatment of previously treated hand infections. J Trauma 1985;25:163–4.

Fingertip Infections

James Barger, MD, Rohit Garg, MBBS, Frederick Wang, MD, Neal Chen, MD*

KEYWORDS

• Fingertip • Infection • Paronychia • Felon • Hand

KEY POINTS

- The fingertip is the most common site of infections in the hand, and these infections frequently are encountered by surgeons, dermatologists, and emergency and primary providers.
- Paronychia are infections of the nail fold that require adequate decompression if an abscess has formed. Acute and chronic forms differ in pathophysiology and treatment.
- Felons are infections of the volar fingertip pulp, a closed anatomic compartment, and can progress to flexor tenosynovitis and osteomyelitis if not managed appropriately.
- Numerous infectious, rheumatologic, and oncologic conditions can mimic these common infections and must be considered by the managing clinician.

INTRODUCTION

The fingertip is the most common site of hand infections.[1,2] Infections of the fingertip may present to hand surgeons, dermatologists, primary care physicians, and emergency physicians. Early diagnosis and treatment are key to minimizing morbidity and disability.[3] Although the management of common hand infections is relatively consistent, recent studies have shed light on optimal treatment. This review seeks to direct clinicians in an evidence-based manner, to make them aware of more obscure conditions that can mimic common infections, and to provide an understanding of the relevant anatomy of the fingertip.

ANATOMY

The fingertip is composed of the distal phalanx, insertion of the terminal extensor and flexor digitorum profundus (FDP) tendons, nail plate and nail bed, volar pad, and the enveloping skin. The fingertip pad is a closed compartment that consists of columns of fat within a supporting lattice of collagen bands, sometimes described as the straps of a parachute, anchoring the skin to the volar periosteum of the distal phalanx.[4] A common misconception is that these bands form discrete compartments.[4]

The fingernail protects the fingertip, regulates temperature, and provides counterpressure for he sensory organs contained therein, enabling fine manipulation.[5] The nail bed attaches to the periosteum of the distal phalanx dorsally and consists of the germinal and sterile matrices. The germinal matrix is deep to the proximal nail fold and produces the majority of the nail plate.[6] It originates 2 mm distal to the extensor insertion as basilar cells and terminates at the lunula; it is more vascular than the sterile matrix. The basilar cells migrate distally as new cells are formed and flatten as they contact the nail plate, leading to longitudinal nail growth. The retention of nuclei in the younger of these cells is what makes that lunula white. The sterile matrix is the nail bed distal to the lunula; it contributes in a minor way (10%) to nail formation. The sterile matrix has linear ridges, which anchor the nail plate, making the nail more adherent to this matrix than the germinal.[6] The term, *paronychium*, refers to the folds of skin on either side of the sterile matrix. The *eponychium* is the soft tissue overlying the proximal nail plate, which extends from the dorsal skin. The

Division of Hand Surgery, Department of Orthopaedic Surgery, Massachusetts General Hospital, MGH Orthopaedic Hand Surgery, Yawkey Center for Outpatient Care, 55 Fruit Street, Suite 2C, Boston, MA 02114-2696, USA
* Corresponding author.
E-mail address: nchen1@partners.org

Hand Clin 36 (2020) 313–321
https://doi.org/10.1016/j.hcl.2020.03.004

hyponychium is a plug of keratinous material at the junction of the distal sterile matrix and the skin, packed with white blood cells, which seals off the subungual space.[5] Perionychium refers to the nail bed, nail plate, and surrounding skin folds collectively.

ACUTE PARONYCHIA
Background and Epidemiology

Infections underlying the paronychium or eponychium are called paronychia. These occur from inoculation of bacteria, often after minor trauma.[7] Paronychia are the most common infections in the hand.[8] Diagnosis is based on history and examination; blood tests usually are unnecessary. If a highly aggressive infection is suspected or an infection has been present for longer than a few days, radiographs may be helpful in identifying bony erosion. Paronychia typically present with 4 days to 5 days of painful swelling and erythema of the paronychium and/or eponychium.[2,9] Subungual infections are uncommon except in those who engage in activities that disrupt the hyponychium, such as dishwashing.[5] A useful examination finding to suggest and localize associated abscess (requiring drainage) is the digital pressure test described by Turkmen and colleagues, in which the skin overlying the abscess blanches and clearly demarcates the abscess cavity with pinch of the fingertip.[10] The interview should include history of exposure to oral secretions or of labial lesions, which might suggest herpetic whitlow; history of rheumatologic and dermatologic conditions that can mimic or predispose to paronychia; and medication history, because several agents are associated with paronychia, as discussed later.[7]

Acute bacterial paronychia are associated with manicures, nail biting, artificial nails, and hangnails (stripping of the paronychium),[11] with onychophagia the most common cause.[2] All these risk factors involve compromise of the nail fold's barrier to infection. Hand infections are more common in immunosuppressed patients.[1,3,11] A recent prospective study found 80% of 103 consecutive acute fingertip infections affected the middle 3 digits, and the eponychium was the most common location (Fig. 1).[2]

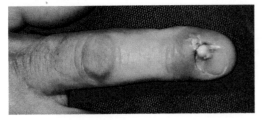

Fig. 1. Acute paronychia.

Microbiology

Published series of fingertip infections consistently find Staphylococcus aureus (SA) the most common offending organism. Rockwell[12] reported that SA, Streptococcus pyogenes, Pseudomonas pyocyanea, and Proteus vulgaris were most common, in order of frequency. Rabarin and colleagues[2] French series of fingertip infections demonstrated 58% SA followed by polymicrobial infection, Streptococcus, and gram-negative rods. Fowler and Ilyas[3] studied 1500 patients undergoing incision and drainage (I&D) of hand infections in an urban center; of the 458 with positive cultures, 53% had methicillin-resistant SA (MRSA), 23% methicillin-sensitive SA, and 19% polymicrobial infection. Polymicrobial infection was strongly associated with diabetes mellitus [DM], intravenous drug use [IVDU], or human bites and should be suspected in these patients).

Treatment

Nonoperative
Early paronychia without abscess formation may be treated with a trial of topical or oral antibiotics. Wollina[13] compared the use of topical gentamicin and topical fusidic acid with betamethasone. Fusidic acid with betamethasone led to symptom improvement in approximately 3 days compared with 5 days for gentamicin.[13] There is some concern, however, that the use of corticosteroids in the setting of an infection may not be advised. Oral antibiotics should cover gram-positive cocci as well as gram negative and anaerobic bacteria in patients with exposure to oral flora or animals (eg, amoxicillin/clavulanate).[3,7,14,15] Empiric coverage for MRSA is recommended in communities with a prevalence of more than 10%. Several investigators advocate water, saline, or antiseptic soaks in conjunction with the modalities discussed previously, although the value of their contribution is unknown and they have not been studied on their own.[1,7,16]

Operative
If an abscess is present or medical treatment is not effective, I&D are recommended. If the abscess is adjacent to the nail fold, it can be opened up by incising the sulcus between the nail fold and the nail.[17] This can be done sharply with a no. 11 or no. 15 scalpel or bluntly with a Freer elevator or hemostat. The blade should be directed away from the nail to avoid injury to the nail bed and subsequent deformity.[7] A 21-gauge or 23-gauge needle also may be used with the bevel directed upward.[18] Gauze packing can facilitate drainage by preventing the skin from prematurely closing over

the wound. The nail plate does not need to be elevated unless there is subungual extension of the abscess, and nail removal generally is reserved for cases in which the infection dissects the nail plate free from the matrix.[7] In cases of subeponychial infection or a runaround infection, parallel dorsal incisions in line with the lateral nail folds allow the eponychium to be reflected proximally to drain the abscess. A variation is the Swiss roll technique, in which the distal end of the eponychium is reflected proximally over gauze and sutured in place for 2 days to 7 days.[7,19] Excision of the eponychium has been described but should be avoided if possible, because this leads to loss of the cells that provide the nail its shine, leading to a dull and irregular nail.[5] Paronychia also may be decompressed with longitudinal incisions, particularly if the abscess is sufficiently large or distant from midline to make drainage through the sulcus difficult, although this poses the risk of necrosis to the resultant skin bridge.[17]

Antibiotics

It is unclear whether antibiotics are needed after I&D. Two recent studies from France suggest that if patients are compliant with prescribed wound care, antibiotics may not be necessary. Pierrart and colleagues[20] treated 46 patients (26 with paronychia, 3 with felon, and 17 with both) with I&D without antibiotics; there was only 1 case of recurrence. Rabarin and colleagues[2] treated 103 fingertip infections with wide "almost oncologic" excision of the affected area: in the 73 felt to have uncomplicated paronychia and not already on antibiotics, no antibiotics were prescribed. Five of these required antibiotic prescriptions at the post-I&D wound check for infection persistence in the setting of noncompliance with wound care; only 1 had infection persistence despite compliance. All infections resolved and wounds healed at routine 1-month check. Regarding closed space infections in general, a systematic review of trials of antibiotics after abscess drainage among 589 patients found that adjuvant antibiotics did not improve rates of abscess resolution.[21]

Wound care

There are few data on optimal wound care, but it may involve wick changes. The guiding principle is that contaminated or saturated dressings should not be maintained in the wound for any prolonged period.

Soaks

Soaks, such as water, saline, povidone-iodine, hydrogen peroxide, and chlorhexidine, are used as an adjunct in many published fingertip infection series. Typically, soaks are recommended for 5 days to 7 days or until symptom resolution.[1,8,14] Unfortunately, none of these studies investigated the role of soaks in a controlled manner. A recently published prospective, randomized trial on povidone-iodine soaks after hand infection I&D (including but not limited to fingertip infections), however, found no benefit from soaks relative to daily gauze dressing changes with regard to the number of débridements required or length of stay, suggesting that soaks may be unnecessary.[22]

CHRONIC PARONYCHIA
Background and Epidemiology

Chronic paronychia exist when inflammation of the nail fold has been present for 6 weeks or more.[7] Erythema and swelling are present but usually not as severe as in acute paronychia.[1] Typically, chronic paronychia occur when a finger is exposed to repetitive mechanical and/or chemical insults that break down the skin.[23] Commonly affected groups include bartenders, homemakers, dishwashers, swimmers, florists, and nurses.[7,17] Beau lines (transverse grooves in the nail plate representing disruption of growth) may be seen and multiple digits usually are involved.[24] DM and immunosuppression increase the risk for chronic paronychia.[7] Certain medications can cause chronic paronychia, including epidermal growth factor receptor inhibitors[14,25] (17% of users), chemotherapeutics such as taxanes (35% of users),[14] antiretrovirals such as indinavir and lamivudine (4% of users),[14,26–28] retinoids,[28] antiepileptics,[29] and methotrexate. These effects usually are due to toxicity to the epithelium, and changes are manifested several weeks after drug administration due to the time it takes for the nail to grow.[29]

Treatment

Candida albicans can be cultured in 40% to 95% of chronic paronychia.[7,14,23,24,30] For this reason, fungal infection was long thought to be a cause of chronic paronychia; however, a randomized, double-blind trial demonstrated that topical steroids are more effective than antifungals at resolving these paronychia, suggesting that fungal presence represents an opportunistic colonization of the inflamed nail fold rather than the underlying cause of inflammation.[30]

The primary treatment of chronic paronychia is irritant avoidance, eliminating the repetitive insult that caused the disease.[7,24] Topical steroids or calcineurin inhibitors address inflammation and are effective treatments.[30] Use of systemic steroids also been has described.[14] Antibiotics have been used as an adjunct to surgical management but may not be necessary unless there is an acute component, with erythema and/or purulence.[24]

Some cases of chronic paronychia do not respond to nonsurgical management. Edema, induration, and fibrosis compromise blood flow and can make spontaneous healing difficult, even with irritant avoidance.[31,32] Marsupialization is a technique in which the proximal nail fold is made to communicate with the external environment by reflection or excision of the eponychium, with or without leaving a rim of tissue distally or removing the nail plate. Numerous investigators have reported success with these methods, although the curative mechanism is not fully understood.[7,31–33] The excision of a crescent of eponychium has been reported as successful both with and without inclusion of the subcutaneous fat, suggesting extension down to the nail may not be necessary.[31,33] Nail plate removal may be helpful in those with nail changes.[33] The Swiss roll technique may be used but for a longer duration than in acute cases (7–14 days instead of 2–7 days).[19]

FELON
Background, Epidemiology, and Microbiology

The term *felon* comes from Old French; the prefix *fel* refers to bile. Thus, a fingertip felon refers to collection of poisonous bile just as a criminal felon refers to a person containing this evil humor.[34] A felon is an infection of the volar pulp of the distal phalanx, typically presenting with erythema, swelling, and pain. As pressure from the infection builds, venous return may be compromised, increasing congestion of the fingertip and leading to tissue necrosis and formation of an abscess.[35] Felons represent 15% to 20% of all hand infections.[36]

The etiology of felon is often unclear.[9,37] Kanavel,[38] in his 1912 description of fingertip anatomy, stated that "the glands lying in the columns of fat present a portal for the entrance of pathogenic bacteria"; perhaps this 100-year-old hypothesis for the etiology of atraumatic felon is correct.[38] Reported causes of felon include glucometer finger sticks, splinters, and disco dancing.[39,40] As with other hand infections, DM is a risk factor.[40] With regard to microbiology, SA is the most common causative agent but felons more likely are polymicrobial in patients with IVDU, DM, farm work, or bites.[41] Eikenella may be seen in diabetic nail-biters (**Figs. 2 and 3**).[42]

Treatment

There is minimal hard evidence on optimal treatment of felon.[40] Namely, it is unclear when

nonoperative management suffices versus when incision is necessary. Bolton and colleagues described felon as having a cellulitic stage, which can be treated medically, and an abscess stage, which requires incision—with the former having a more "prickly" pain and the latter more "throbbing."[9] The decision for incision often is made based on clinical judgment and experience. It has been argued that incision should be made when the skin of the distal phalanx is tense, whether or not there is an abscess, to relieve vascular congestion in the fingertip.[35] If nonoperative management with antibiotics and elevation is to be trialed, appropriate antibiotics should be chosen to cover gram-positive cocci, with coverage of MRSA and other pathogens included if there is reasonable suspicion of their involvement. Patients should be followed closely to determine need for progression to I&D.

Inadequate treatment of felon can have dire consequences; reported complications of neglect include skin slough, ischemia/necrosis of the surrounding structures (fingertip compartment syndrome), osteomyelitis, septic arthritis, flexor tenosynovitis, and flexor tendon rupture. Osteomyelitis, flexor tenosynovitis, and tendon rupture have been described as the triad of neglected felon.[37] Watson and Jebson[37] described an IVDU with DM who presented with these sequelae 18 days after felon symptom onset; he required amputation through the interphalangeal joint, then later the metacarpophalangeal joint in addition to tendon sheath I&D. Felons can decompress through several routes—a sinus tract to the skin or through the nail fold to form a paronychia—or invade from periosteum to bone and to tendon sheath. Presence of a sinus warrants radiographs to evaluate for possible osteomyelitis. In some cases, pus may decompress through the dermis but not the epidermis, dissecting in this layer.[9] Felons typically do not spread proximally in the subcutaneous tissue due to the attachment of joint crease to deep fascia, which creates a closed compartment (**Fig. 4**).[35]

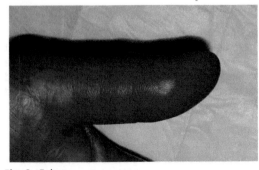

Fig. 2. Felon.

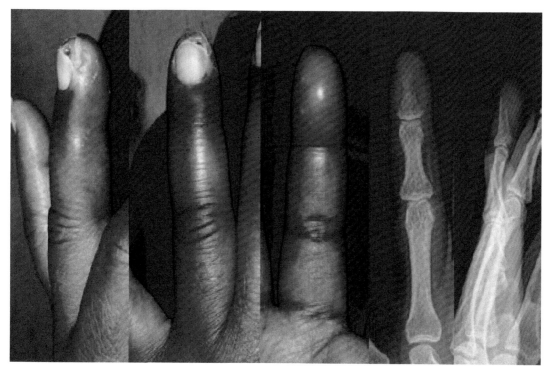

Fig. 3. Felon with associated osteomyelitis, which required amputation.

The mainstay of felon management is I&D. Some investigators advocate using a midlateral J-shaped incision on the noncontact side of the fingertip to avoid the volar pad and prevent devascularization of dorsal skin; other investigators argue for incision right over the area of fluctuance, given risk of digital nerve injury and resultant causalgia in lateral incisions.[9,35,43] Fishmouth incisions may pose a risk of soft tissue necrosis.[43] The authors prefer an incision located directly over the area of maximum fluctuance or skin tension. If a sinus is present, it should be excised with an ellipse of tissue. Inadvertent penetration of the tendon sheath can cause flexor tenosynovitis, which may be a reason to avoid aggressive proximal probing.[9] The authors usually place a wick and continue wick changes for 2 days to 5 days to allow continued drainage.[43]

The conventional view of felon anatomy, first advanced by Koch[44] in 1929 and advocated in much of the literature, is that the collagen bands of the volar pulp constitute septae, forming microcompartments that render simple I&D inadequate for infection control unless they are broken up.[44] This compartment theory is controversial, however, and some investigators suggest simple decompression.[4,35] That said, abscesses elsewhere in the body form loculations that must be broken up during drainage and, if present, should be addressed in the fingertip as well.[45]

MIMICS

There are numerous oncologic, rheumatologic, and infectious conditions that may mimic the infections discussed previously, in particular paronychia. Knowledge is important because their management is different from that of paronychia or felon, involving oncologic resection for malignancies and medical therapy for rheumatologic conditions and infectious mimics. These diagnoses should be considered particularly in cases that do not respond to antibiotics or drainage. A Turkish group performed cytology on a series of 58 patients with presumptive diagnoses of paronychia who had not responded to antibiotics; only 43% of these infections were bacterial. Of those, 19% were herpetic and 17% were parapox (orf) virus; other etiologies included fungal infections, drug reactions, and pemphigus vulgaris.[46] Although cytology may not be available routinely and usually is unnecessary, these reports illustrate the need to be aware of the differential diagnosis, particularly in cases that do not respond to treatment.

Calcific Tendinitis/Periarthritis

Calcific tendinitis/periarthritis is the deposition of calcium hydroxyapatite in tendon substance or ligaments/capsule around the joint. It is seen more commonly in the shoulder and is rare in

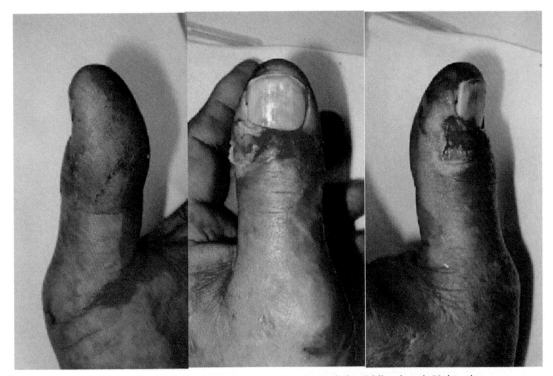

Fig. 4. Felon that has decompressed as a paronychia. Left: volar-radial, Middle: dorsal, Right: ulnar.

the hand; however, reports have described involvement of the FDP and the distal interphalangeal (DIP) joint.[47,48] In the fingertip, it can present as acute onset of pain, swelling, and erythema with elevated inflammatory markers and can mimic a felon, septic arthritis of DIP, or flexor tenosynovitis. Radiographs may show calcific deposition (**Fig. 5**). It is a self-limiting process and treatment with anti-inflammatory medication, oral steroids, or corticosteroid injection is effective.[47]

Gout

Gout is the inflammatory response to deposition of monosodium urate crystals. Gout can involve the DIP joints and acute tophaceous gout can mimic felon, paronychia, and DIP septic arthritis. Acute tophus can present with a red, hot, and swollen fingertip and liquid tophus can mimic purulent discharge.[49] Radiographs may demonstrate underlying arthritic changes in the joint with periarticular erosions. Medical management with nonsteroidal anti-inflammatory drugs and/or colchicine usually is effective.

Herpetic Whitlow

Herpetic whitlow is the term for herpes simplex virus (types 1 and 2) infections of the pulp of the distal phalanx; the rest of the hand may be involved as

well. Its incidence is 2.5 per 100,000 individuals.[50] Dentists, dental hygienists, hairdressers, and health care workers traditionally are at risk via occupational exposure to oral secretions; however, the routine use of gloves has decreased transmission by this route. The disease is common in children who suck their thumbs and can occur in the feet as well.[50] It is characterized by painful erythematous and vesicular eruptions. These are extremely contagious during the first 2 weeks.[50] Late in the infection, white blood cells may deposit in the lesion, but there is never frank purulence in herpetic whitlow unless there is a bacterial superinfection.[50] The disease is self-limiting over a 3-week to 4-week course. No incision is recommended because of risk of superinfection.[46,51] Oral acyclovir should be prescribed in equivalent doses to oral/genital infections.[50]

Cancer

Numerous malignancies have been reported as mimicking paronychia by manifesting in or adjacent to the nail bed. These include squamous cell carcinoma/Bowen disease, melanoma, Kaposi sarcoma, papillary adenocarcinoma, and amyloidosis.[52–57] An apparent isolated chronic paronychia when all other nails are healthy should raise concern for a malignancy.[14,24] Chronic immunosuppression also should raise suspicion.[56]

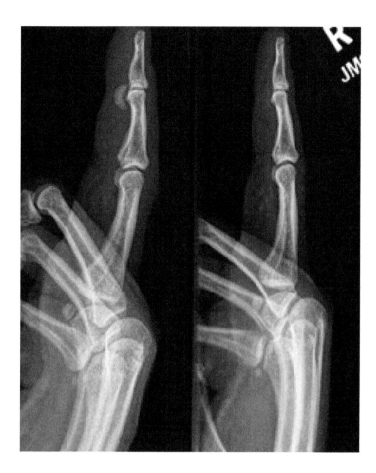

Fig. 5. Radiographs demonstrating calcific tendonitis of the FDP insertion and resolution after nonsteroidal anti-inflammatory drug course. Left: Before NSAIDs; Right: After NSAIDs.

Treatment of these lesions varies by diagnosis but generally begins with tissue diagnosis.

Autoimmune Conditions

Several rheumatologic conditions can cause nail changes. These may be suspected based on the presence of systemic lesions characteristic of that disease.

- Psoriasis: nail pitting and oil spots, characteristic scaly skin lesions
- Reactive arthritis: Reiter triad—conjunctivitis, urethritis, and arthritis
- Pemphigus vulgaris: oral, cutaneous, and conjunctival lesions[58]

Zoonoses

There are several less common fingertip infections that may be found in those having contact with animals. Orf disease is caused by parapox virus and is found most commonly in individuals who interact with sheep or goats. It presents with a painful wheal on the fingertip, 2 cm to 3 cm in diameter, with clear exudate. It may cause systemic fever and malaise, particularly in immunocompromised patients.[50] It is a self-limiting disease lasting 6 weeks to 8 weeks and, like herpetic whitlow, should not be treated with incision.[59] Similar to orf disease and grouped with it under the classification of farmyard pox is milker nodule, a 0.5-cm to 2-cm erythematous nodule found in those exposed to infected cows.[50]

Cat bites may cause serious infection and most commonly affect the hand and fingertips. As opposed to dog bites, which tend to cause significant soft tissue destruction and open wounds, the sharp and narrow teeth of cats may inoculate bacteria deeply without disruption of the overlying soft tissues.[60] *Pasteurella multocida* is a gram-negative coccobacillus that is the most common pathogen in these bites and is well covered by amoxicillin-clavulanate. Evaluation should include assessment of erythema, drainage, fluctuance, and pain with joint range of motion concerning for a joint or tendon sheath infection. Management depends on the severity of presentation, but if outpatient management is trialed, follow-up should be close, because 30% require hospital admission, the majority of which undergoes surgical débridement.[60]

Erysipeloid (of Rosenbach) is a bacterial infection caused by *Erysipelothrix rhusiopathiae* and caused by trauma to the hand experienced while handling lobsters, livestock, meat, and so forth. It is characterized by an inflammatory red-purple lesion and there may be vesicular eruption and erosions. It is sensitive to most antibiotics.[61]

Sporothrix schenckii

The dimorphic fungus *Sporothrix schenckii* also may affect the fingertip. Sporotrichosis is common in gardeners and occurs days to weeks after the skin is inoculated with the fungus, stereotypically after sticking a finger on a thorn. A nodule develops that typically ulcerates and drains nonpurulent fluid. The infection spreads proximally via lymphatics with additional lesions appearing along these tracts.[62] It is treated with itraconazole for 3 months to 6 months.[63]

DISCLOSURE

The authors have nothing to disclose.

REFERENCES

1. Jebson P. Infections of the fingertip. Paronychias and felons. Hand Clin 1998;14(4):547–55.
2. Rabarin F, Jeudy J, Cesari B, et al. Acute finger-tip infection: Management and treatment. A 103-case series. Orthop Traumatol Surg Res 2017;103(6):933–6.
3. Fowler J, Ilyas A. Epidemiology of adult acute hand infections at an urban medical center. J Hand Surg Am 2013;38(6):1189–93.
4. Hauck R, Camp L, Ehrlich H, et al. Pulp nonfiction: microscopic anatomy of the digital pulp space. Plast Reconstr Surg 2004;113(2):536–9.
5. Zook EG. Anatomy and physiology of the perionychium. Clin Anat 2003;16(1):1–8.
6. Zook E. Anatomy and physiology of the perionychium. Hand Clin 1990;6(1):1–7.
7. Shafritz A, Coppage J. Acute and chronic paronychia of the hand. J Am Acad Orthop Surg 2014;22(3):165–74.
8. Ritting AW, O'Malley MP, Rodner CM. Acute paronychia. J Hand Surg Am 2012;37(5):1068–70.
9. Bolton H, Fowler PJ, Jepson RP. Natural history and treatment of pulp space infection and osteomyelitis of the terminal phalanx. J Bone Joint Surg Br 1949;31B:499–504.
10. Turkmen A, Warnter R, Page R. Digital pressure test for paronychia. Br J Plast Surg 2004;57(1):93–4.
11. Franko OI, Abrams RA. Hand infections. Orthop Clin North Am 2013;44(4):625–34.
12. Rockwell P. Acute and chronic paronychia. Am Fam Physician 2001;63:1113–36.
13. Wollina U. Acute paronychia: Comparative treatment with topical antibiotic alone or in combination with corticosteroid. J Eur Acad Dermatol Venereol 2001;15(1):82–4.
14. Rigopoulos D, Larios G, Gregoriou S, et al. Acute and chronic paronychia. Am Fam Physician 2008;77(3):339–46.
15. Tosti R, Ilyas A. Empiric antibiotics for acute infections of the hand. J Hand Surg Am 2010;35(1):125–8.
16. Daniel CI. Paronychia. Dermatol Clin 1985;3(3):461–4.
17. Canales F, Newmeyer WI, Kilgore EJ. The treatment of felons and paronychias. Hand Clin 1989;5(4):515–23.
18. Ogunlusi J, Oginni L, Ogunlusi O. DAREJD simple technique of draining acute paronychia. Tech Hand Up Extrem Surg 2005;9(2):120–1.
19. Pabari A, Iyer S, Khoo C. Swiss roll technique for treatment of paronychia. Tech Hand Up Extrem Surg 2011;15(2):75–7.
20. Pierrart J, Delgrande D, Mamane W, et al. Acute felon and paronychia: Antibiotics not necessary after surgical treatment. Prospective study of 46 patients. Hand Surg Rehabil 2016;35(1):40–3.
21. Singer A, Thode HJ. Systemic antibiotics after incision and drainage of simple abscesses: a meta-analysis. Emerg Med J 2014;31(4):576–8.
22. Tosti R, Iorio J, Fowler J, et al. Povidone-iodine soaks for hand abscesses: a prospective randomized trial. J Hand Surg Am 2014;39(5):962–5.
23. Daniel CI, Daniel M, Daniel C, et al. Chronic paronychia and onycholysis: A thirteen-year experience. Cutis 1996;58(6):397–401.
24. Leggit JC. Acute and chronic paronychia. Am Fam Physician 2017;96(1):44–51.
25. Dianichi T, Tanaka M, Tsuruta N, et al. Development of multiple paronychia and periungual granulation in patients treated with gefitinib, an inhibitor of epidermal growth factor receptor. Dermatology 2003;207(3):324–5.
26. Tosti A, Piraccini B, D'Antuono A, et al. Paronychia associated with antiretroviral therapy. Br J Dermatol 1999;140(6):1165–8.
27. Daudén E, Pascual-López M, Martinez-García C, et al. Paronychia and excess granulation tissue of the toes and finger in a patient treated with indinavir. Br J Dermatol 2000;142(5):1063–4.
28. Sass J, Jakob-Sölder B, Heitger A, et al. Paronychia with pyogenic granuloma in a child treated with indinavir: The retinoid-mediated side effect theory revisited. Dermatology 2000;200(1):40–2.
29. Hardin J, Haber R, Onychomadesis. literature review. Br J Dermatol 2015;172(3):592–6.
30. Tosti A, Piraccini B, Ghetti E, et al. Topical steroids versus systemic antifungals in the treatment of chronic paronychia: An open, randomized double-

blind and double dummy study. J Am Acad Dermatol 2002;47(1):73–6.

31. Keyser J, Eaton R. Surgical cure of chronic paronychia by eponychial marsupialization. Plast Reconstr Surg 1976;58(1):66–70.

32. Grover C, Bansal S, Nanda S, et al. En bloc excision of proximal nail fold for treatment of chronic paronychia. Dermatol Surg 2006;32(3):393–9.

33. Bednar M, Lane L. Eponychial marsupialization and nail removal for surgical treatment of chronic paronychia. J Hand Surg Am 1991;16(2):314–7.

34. Diab M. Lexicon of orthopaedic etymology. Amsterdam (the Netherlands): Harwood Academic Publishers; 1999.

35. Kilgore EJ, Brown L, Newmeyer W, et al. Treatment of felons. Am J Surg 1975;130(2):194–8.

36. Linscheid R, Dobyns J. Common and uncommon infections of the hand. Orthop Clin North Am 1975;6: 1063–104.

37. Watson PA, Jebson PJ. The natural history of the neglected felon. Iowa Orthop J 1996;16:164–6.

38. Kanavel A. Infection of the hand. New York: The Classics of Surgery Library, division of Gryphon Editions; 1992.

39. Walker F, Lillemoe K, Farquharson R. Disco felon. N Engl J Med 1979;301(3):166–7.

40. Tannan SC, Deal DN. Diagnosis and management of the acute felon: evidence-based review. J Hand Surg Am 2012;37(12):2603–4.

41. Abrams RA, Botte MJ. Hand infections: treatment recommendations for specific types. J Am Acad Orthop Surg 1996;4(4):219–30.

42. Imahara SD, Friedrich JB. Community-acquired methicillin-resistant Staphylococcus aureus in surgically treated hand infections. J Hand Surg Am 2010;35A.

43. Stevanovic MV, Sharpe F. Acute infections of the hand. In: Wolfe SW, Hotchkiss RN, Pederson WC, et al, editors. Green's operative hand surgery. 7th edition. Philadelphia: Elsevier; 2017. p. 17–61.

44. Koch SL. Felons: Acute lymphangitis and tendon sheath infections. JAMA 1929;92(14):1171–3.

45. Meislin H, McGehee M, Rosen P. Management and microbiology of cutaneous abscesses. JACEP 1978;7(5):186–91.

46. Durdu M, Ruocco V. Clinical and cytologic features of antibiotic-resistant acute paronychia. J Am Acad Dermatol 2014;70(1):120–6.

47. Kim J, Lee J, Park J, et al. Acute Calcific Tendinitis in the Distal Interphalangeal Joint. Arch Plast Surg 2016;43(3):301–3.

48. Munjal A, Munjal P, Mahajan A. Diagnostic dilemma: acute calcific tendinitis of flexor digitorum profundus. Hand (N Y) 2013;8(3):352–3.

49. Fitzgerald B, Setty A, Mudgal C. Gout affecting the hand and wrist. J Am Acad Orthop Surg 2007; 15(10):625–35.

50. Adisen E, Onder M. Acral manifestations of viral infections. Clin Dermatol 2017;35(1):40–9.

51. Szinnai G, Schaad U, Heininger U. Multiple herpetic whitlow lesions in a 4-year-old girl: Case report and review of the literature. Eur J Pediatr 2001;160: 528–33.

52. Gorva A, Mohil R, Srinivasan M. Aggressive digital papillary adenocarcinoma presenting as a paronychia of the finger. J Hand Surg Br 2005;30(5):534.

53. Keith J, Wilgis E. Kaposi's sarcoma in the hand of an AIDS patient. J Hand Surg Am 1986;11(3):410–3.

54. Ahmed I, Cronk J, Crutchfield CI, et al. Myeloma-associated systemic amyloidosis presenting as chronic paronychia and palmodigital erythematous swelling and induration of the hands. J Am Acad Dermatol 2000;42(2 part 2):339–42.

55. Ware J. Sub-ungual malignant melanoma presenting as sub-acute paronychia following trauma. Hand 2010;9(1):49–51.

56. Fung V, Sainsbury D, Seukeran D, et al. Squamous cell carcinoma of the finger masquerading as paronychia. J Plast Reconstr Aesthet Surg 2010;63(2):e191–2.

57. Bryant J, Gardner P, Yousif M, et al. Aggressive Digital Papillary Adenocarcinoma of the Hand Presenting as a Felon. Case Rep Orthop 2017;2017: 6456342.

58. Engineer L, Norton L, Ahmed A. Nail involvement in pemphigus vulgaris. J Am Acad Dermatol 2000; 43(3):529–35.

59. Arnaud J, Bernard P, Souyri N, et al. Human ORF disease localized in the hand: a "false felon". A study of eight cases. Ann Chir Main 1986;5(2):129–32.

60. Babovic N, Cayci C, Carlsen B. Cat bite infections of the hand: assessment of morbidity and predictors of severe infection. J Hand Surg Am 2014;39(2): 286–90.

61. Veraldi S, Girgenti V, Dassoni F, et al. Erysipeloid: a review. Clin Exp Dermatoal 2009;34(8):859–62.

62. Barros M, de Almeida Paes R, Schubach A. Sporothrix schenckii and Sporotrichosis. Clin Microbiol Rev 2011;24(4):633–54.

63. Sharkey-Mathis P, Kauffman C, Graybill J, et al. Treatment of sporotrichosis with itraconazole. NIAID Mycoses Study Group. Am J Med 1993;95(3): 279–85.

Pyogenic Flexor Tenosynovitis: Evaluation and Management

Kanu Goyal, MD*, Amy L. Speeckaert, MD, MS

KEYWORDS

• Flexor tenosynovitis • Pyogenic • Suppurative • Finger infection

KEY POINTS

- Pyogenic flexor tenosynovitis is an infection of the flexor tendon sheath that should be managed urgently to prevent propagation to other digits, the carpal tunnel, and the distal forearm.
- Diagnosis of pyogenic flexor tenosynovitis is typically accomplished with a thorough history and physical examination, looking especially for the 4 Kanavel signs: diffuse finger swelling, finger held in a flexed posture, pain with passive digital extension, and tenderness along the flexor tendon sheath.
- *Staphylococcus aureus* is the most common species involved in pyogenic flexor tenosynovitis, although several other species may be involved, especially in immunocompromised individuals.
- Closed tendon sheath irrigation has become the standard of care for pyogenic flexor tenosynovitis.
- Early postoperative finger range of motion is encouraged to help prevent prolonged finger stiffness.

INTRODUCTION

Pyogenic flexor tenosynovitis (PFT) is a closed-space infection of the flexor tendon sheath system of the fingers, thumb, or hand. Interconnections between the individual tendon sheaths, known as the radial, ulnar, and palmar bursa, allow rapid spread of infection throughout the hand.[1] Early diagnosis and treatment remain critical, because persistent infection can lead to permanent loss of hand function. The pathophysiology of flexor tenosynovitis was first described by Dr Allen B. Kanavel,[1] who recognized its ability to produce a devastating outcome when not treated early in its course. In 1 study, its prevalence was reported to be as high as 9.4% of all hand infections.[2] Prompt diagnosis and appropriate treatment are essential to prevent spread of infection and preserve hand function.

RELEVANT ANATOMY

The finger flexor tendon sheath is thought to be a closed anatomic space with an inner visceral layer and an outer parietal layer. The synovial space between the layers can become distended under pressure with an infection. The relatively avascular nature of the tendon sheaths and hand bursae provides an ideal environment for bacteria to propagate without recognition by the host's immune system. Each finger contains 5 annular (A1–A5) and 3 cruciate (C1–C3) pulleys (**Fig. 1**), whereas the thumb contains 3 annular pulleys (A1, A2, and the annular variable pulley) and 1 oblique pulley. A2 and A4 pulleys in the fingers and the oblique pulley in the thumb are thought to be required to prevent bowstringing and should be preserved, if possible, during a surgical debridement of the finger.[3]

Department of Orthopaedic Surgery, Hand & Upper Extremity Center, The Ohio State Wexner Medical Center, 915 Olentangy River Road, Suite 3200, Columbus, OH 43212, USA
* Corresponding author.
E-mail address: Kanu.goyal@osumc.edu

Hand Clin 36 (2020) 323–329
https://doi.org/10.1016/j.hcl.2020.03.005
0749-0712/20/© 2020 Elsevier Inc. All rights reserved.

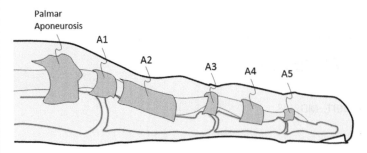

Fig. 1. Finger flexor tendon pulley anatomy.

The tendon sheath of the flexor pollicis longus communicates directly with the radial bursa, whereas the flexor tendon sheath of the small finger (and at times that of the index, middle, and ring fingers) often communicates directly with the ulnar bursa. When the tendon sheath of the digit does not communicate with the ulnar bursa, it typically lies just proximal to the A1 pulley.[2] **(Fig. 2)** shows the most common variation in bursa anatomy (72% of cases). However, in 17% of cases, there may not be any connection between the individual fingers and the ulnar bursa, and in the remaining 11% of cases there are variable interconnections between the fingers and the ulnar bursa.[2] The radial and ulnar bursa communicate with one another in the Parona space (the potential space between the flexor tendons and pronator quadratus in the volar distal forearm), and therefore can give rise to a horseshoe abscess, in which a PFT originating in the thumb causes an infection in the carpal tunnel and in the small finger, or vice-versa. The multiple potential communications between the digits allow the rapid spread of infection from a single puncture wound in one digit to the entire hand, palm, and wrist.[3]

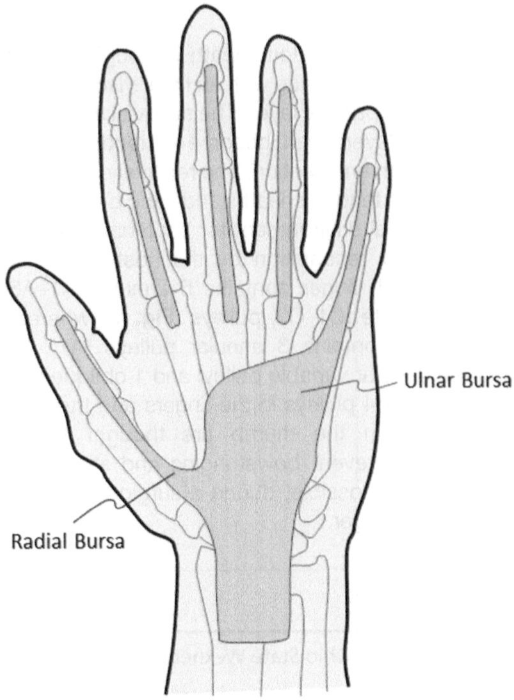

INFECTIOUS EPIDEMIOLOGY

Although the cause of PFT is not always clear, it often originates from inoculation of the flexor tendon sheath as a result of a traumatic wound, puncture, or retained foreign body. However, in many cases, a clear traumatic history is not present and PFT may have occurred secondary to hematogenous seeding.[4,5]

The most commonly isolated organism in patients with PFT is *Staphylococcus aureus*, accounting for 80% of cases. In recent years, methicillin-resistant *S aureus* (MRSA) has been diagnosed with more frequency.[6] *Streptococcus* species and *Pseudomonas aeruginosa* are the next 2 most common species to be cultured. However, it is imperative to recognize that other pathogens may be responsible to ensure effective, targeted antibiotic therapy. In the setting of animal or human bites, *Pasteurella multocida* and *Eikenella corrodens* must be considered, respectively.[7] Immunocompromised patients are at risk for several less common bacteria, such as *Streptococcus mitis*, a strain of *Streptococcus viridans*,[8] as well as gram-negative organisms or mixed flora. Inoculations in marine environments have led to infections from less common pathogens, such as *Mycobacterium marinum* and *Shewanella algae*.[9,10] Even more rare species have been isolated from the flexor tendon sheath, such as *Nocardia nova*, a gram-positive, acid-fast filamentous bacterium that is better known as a cause of pulmonary infections.[11]

Fig. 2. The most common variations of finger flexor tendon sheath anatomy and their communications with the radial and ulnar bursa.

CLINICAL PRESENTATION
History

The most common symptom is pain. Often, the pain is exquisite, particularly with any active or passive motion of the digit. Patients may recall a penetrating injury that occurred days before the onset of symptoms, although many patients deny any such injury. In 1 study, 76% of patients diagnosed with PFT reported a history of recent trauma to the digit. Only 61% of patients reported a known penetrating wound, and 11% reported a blunt trauma without a known source of tendon sheath innoculation.[12]

Symptom progression typically occurs from mild to severe within 1 to 3 days, although in atypical infections it may extend over a longer period of time. Patients may also complain of finger swelling, stiffness, and poor hand function. In cases where there was a penetrating injury, the patient may also complain of drainage, sometimes purulent. PFT can also occur postoperatively, such as after a flexor tendon repair or a trigger finger release. Systemic symptoms of infection may also be present, such as fevers or general malaise, especially in instances where several digits may be involved or an associated abscess may be present. Patients who are immunocompromised are more susceptible to developing PFT after a penetrating injury, surgery, or even atraumatically. They are also more likely to develop complications associated with PFT, such as abscesses or tissue necrosis. A thorough history of comorbidities (diabetes mellitus with or without associated complications, cancer, inflammatory disease, and other potential immunocompromised states) should be elicited. A history of intravenous drug use should also be elicited because this patient population is at risk of PFT caused not only by a possible penetrating needle injury but also by malnutrition. In addition, a thorough list of the patient's current medications should be gathered to look for possible sources of immunosuppression.

Physical Examination

The morbidity of a missed PFT should make it a diagnosis that is assumed present until proved otherwise. The physical examination of a patient with suspected PFT should initially focus on ruling out other explanations for the patient's presenting symptoms. Although systemic infection is not common with isolated PFT, vital signs should be obtained and the patient's general appearance should be assessed. Pang and colleagues[12] noted that only 17% of patients with PFT presented with a fever and none of the 75 patients studied had other systemic signs of infection, such as hypotension or tachycardia. The upper extremity examination should begin with evaluation of the entire arm to look for signs of infection that may have spread more proximally. Cellulitis of the hand or forearm, or a more proximal abscess, may be present. In cases of PFT, special attention should be given to the volar distal forearm at the site of the Parona space, because this area can develop an abscess from proximal tracking of bacteria through the radial or ulnar bursa. Evaluation for possible septic arthritis of the wrist and other small joints of the hand should also be performed because this can penetrate through soft tissues and violate the joint capsule.

Initially described in 1912, Kanavel[13] 4 signs remain the primary tool to diagnose PFT. The presence of exquisite tenderness to palpation of the flexor tendon sheath, a resting flexed posture of the digit, pain with attempted extension of the finger, and fusiform swelling are said to confirm the diagnosis[13] (**Fig. 3**). However, many patients do not present with all 4 signs. Pang and colleagues[12] noted that fusiform swelling was the most common of the signs, with 97% of patients showing this finding. Pain on passive extension was present in 72% of patients, whereas a flexed resting posture of the digit was noted in 69% of patients. Tenderness along the flexor tendon sheath was the least common sign, with 64% complaining of this finding. Dailiana and colleagues[14] found that only 54% (22 out of 41) of patients diagnosed with PFT had all 4 of the Kanavel signs. In pediatric patients, Kanavel signs are less commonly present. Brusalis and colleagues[15]

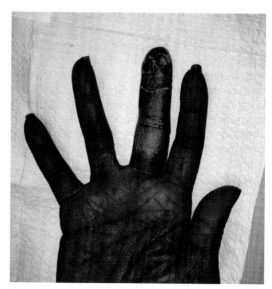

Fig. 3. A patient who had developed pyogenic flexor tenosynovitis of the middle finger.

showed that at least 3 signs were present in 62% of patients, and all 4 signs were present in 34% of pediatric patients. In 3 children, 0 to 1 Kanavel sign was present. Further studies are needed to elucidate the positive predictive value of these criteria based on which and how many signs are present.

Ancillary Studies

Radiographs of the infected digit and hand should be obtained to look for any underlying fractures, retained foreign bodies, arthritic changes, chronic changes suggestive of osteomyelitis, or inflammatory or crystalline arthropathy. When pain and swelling track proximally, radiographs of the wrist should be obtained as well. A recent study comparing radiographs of the finger in patients with PFT and those with non-PFT infected digits concluded that acute PFT swelling is distinguished by volar greater than dorsal soft tissue swelling at the level of the proximal interphalangeal joint.[16] Ultrasonography has also been described as a method to diagnose PFT. A unilateral increase of more than 20% in diameter of the flexor tendon sheath at the level of the A2 pulley was found to predict the diagnosis of PFT and was shown to be reproducible among examiners.[17] Although not routinely used for infections isolated to the finger, MRI is useful to confirm the presence of deep abscesses in the palm as well as to evaluate the proximal extent of soft tissue infection. This method may be particularly useful if physical examination is suggestive of communication of infection between the radial and ulnar bursa in the Parona space.

A complete blood count with differential, erythrocyte sedimentation rate (ESR), and C-reactive protein (CRP) may also be obtained. Although ESR and CRP are nonspecific markers of inflammation, increases in both ESR and CRP level should increase the clinician's suspicion for infection, an inflammatory state. CRP is a useful marker to confirm clinical improvement as the level trends downward. Preoperative laboratory tests are often obtained simultaneously because, when confirmed, PFT is an urgent surgical condition.

Differential Diagnoses

Several conditions present in a similar fashion to PFT, making its diagnosis difficult at times. The differential diagnoses include, but are not limited to, abscess, cellulitis, septic arthritis, gouty arthropathy, aseptic tenosynovitis, a locked trigger finger, and herpetic whitlow.[18] It is imperative to consider the presence of more than 1 diagnosis in any given patient. For example, it is common for a patient to

have PFT, an abscess, ascending cellulitis, and a septic proximal interphalangeal joint.

TREATMENT

Much of the early guidance available for treatment of PFT originated when antibiotics were not available; therefore, the only acceptable treatment was surgical debridement and irrigation. More recently, with the advent of readily available intravenous antibiotics, medical treatment of early PFT has been suggested. Although little evidence is available to support the idea of antibiotics alone for the treatment of PFT,[19,20] the idea has recently gained traction. According to a recent survey of hand surgeons, some are using this tactic in the treatment of what they deem to be early PFT.[21] If symptomatic improvement is not seen within 48 hours or if symptoms worsen, operative management is recommended. Initial antibiotic selection should include presumptive coverage against the most common pathogens, namely MRSA, and should also cover gram-negative rods and anaerobes, especially in immunocompromised patients. Depending on the patient population and specific host, this may include intravenous vancomycin and piperacillin/tazobactam.

Although some surgeons treat clinically mild PFT with intravenous antibiotics, almost all surgeons agree that, in cases of moderate or severe PFT, prompt irrigation of the flexor tendon sheath is indicated.[19] Most surgeons take these patients to the operating room, although the authors have performed successful closed flexor tendon sheath irrigation in the emergency department. Local anesthesia with or without sedation is recommended in single-digit involvement; however, in cases of more extensive infection, such as a horseshoe abscess, general anesthesia may be warranted.

Numerous methods of flexor tendon sheath irrigation have been described, although the concept remains the same: open the closed space and irrigate the tendon sheath, thereby removing the offending agent and decreasing the bacterial load. A survey of hand surgeons in 2019 confirmed the large variation of surgical management. Surgical approach varied greatly, although 77% of respondents advocate 1 incision proximal at the level of the A1 pulley and 1 distal at the level of the A5 pulley, with irrigation using a narrow catheter.[21] The incision distally may be in the distal interphalangeal (DIP) flexor crease or may be a midlateral incision. Various catheters have been used, including angiocatheters (16–22 gauge) and pediatric feeding tubes (4–8 French). Intraluminal wires may be used in feeding tubes to increase the stiffness of the catheter during insertion into the tendon sheath.[22] Modification of the catheters can also be performed to potentially improve irrigation of the tendon sheath, such as by fenestrating the catheter or tube along its length.[19] Haines and McCann[4] describe using a lacrimal probe instead of a feeding tube for irrigation of the sheath, citing the rounded tip and malleability of the probe as advantages compared with the beveled edge and significant flexibility of the feeding tube. Various irrigants, including normal saline alone or with local antibiotics, have been used, showing good outcomes.[4,23]

Although an open debridement with zig-zag or long midaxial incisions was considered the gold standard, closed-catheter irrigation has gained much popularity and perhaps has become the new treatment standard for most cases of PFT. Gutowski and colleagues[23] compared outcomes between open drainage and closed-sheath catheter irrigation through 1 proximal and 1 distal incision and noted, although not statistically significant, a higher complication rate with open drainage. Of note, reexploration was required in 4 out of 32 patients who underwent open drainage and none of the 15 patients that underwent closed-catheter irrigation. Born and colleagues[24] reported on outcomes following both open and closed-catheter irrigation and found similar outcomes with regard to pain, function, and need for reoperation. Nevertheless, an extensive approach with open debridement may still be warranted in cases of severe PFT where tendon necrosis, abscesses, or septic arthritis are present.

Animal studies have evaluated the benefit of locally administered corticosteroids and antibiotics, without surgical drainage, for the treatment of PFT. To date, no human studies have been published, and future studies are warranted before initiating this treatment in humans.[22,25]

POSTOPERATIVE MANAGEMENT

Lille and colleagues[26] compared intraoperative closed-catheter irrigation alone versus intraoperative and continuous postoperative catheter irrigation and found no difference in the complication rate between the two groups, suggesting that intraoperative irrigation alone is sufficient to resolve PFT.

Empiric postoperative antibiotics are initiated and are narrowed based on intraoperative cultures. As noted previously, antibiotic coverage based on the suspected cause of inoculation is critical. With the reported recent increase in prevalence of MRSA in hand infections, strong consideration should be given for empiric coverage.[6]

Other risk factors, such as exposure to animal or human saliva or atypical fungi in known geographic regions, should prompt targeted antibiotic regimens. In addition, consultation with an infectious disease expert should be considered in select cases.

Postoperative protocols with respect to the need for immobilization vary greatly. The need for postoperative splinting and when to initiate motion is debated. Although some clinicians recommend splinting in the intrinsic safe position during the immediate postoperative period,[23,24,27] others recommend immediate postoperative range of motion.[27,28]

AUTHOR'S PREFERRED TREATMENT METHOD

The authors have a low threshold to operate on PFT and rarely manage PFT with intravenous antibiotics alone. We prefer closed tendon sheath irrigation using a longitudinal or oblique incision at the level of the A1 pulley and a transverse incision at the DIP flexion crease. **Figs. 4** and **5** show our standard technique. Although the entire A5 pulley is incised, only the proximal half of the A1 pulley is incised, making insertion of an angiocatheter easier through the intact distal half of the A1 pulley (at the conclusion of the surgery, the remaining portion of A1 is released). After cultures are taken, an 18-gauge angiocatheter is passed antegrade through the A1 pulley and held in place with a hemostat. Several 20-mL syringes with normal saline are used to irrigate the finger flexor tendon sheath. Allowing the digit to gently flex at the proximal interphalangeal (PIP) and DIP crease helps allow smooth irrigation through the tendon sheath and out of the A5 pulley. Confirmation of irrigant flow out of the A5 pulley distally is important to avoid pressurizing the irrigant into the subcutaneous

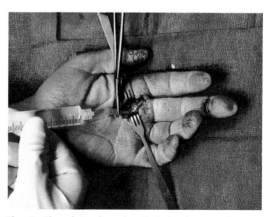

Fig. 4. Closed tendon sheath irrigation can be performed with a proximal incision at the A1 pulley and a distal incision at the A5 pulley.

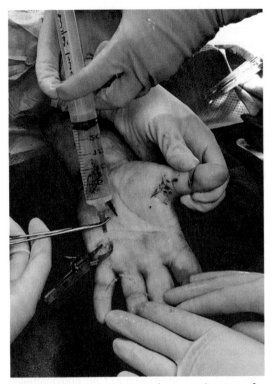

Fig. 5. A patient who went to the operating room for closed tendon sheath irrigation of the thumb, small finger, and carpal tunnel/Parona space. Patient had a puncture wound over his small finger and subsequently developed a horseshoe abscess.

tissues of the digit. In cases where additional subcutaneous abscesses or PIP joint septic arthritis is suspected, midaxial incisions or zig-zag incisions are made (**Fig. 6**). If irrigant is visualized to seep out of the flexor tendon sheath causing global finger swelling, midaxial incisions are helpful to vent the soft tissues to decrease swelling and aid

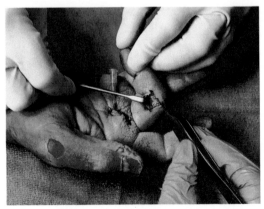

Fig. 6. A midaxial incision can be made to evacuate a subcutaneous finger abscess or septic PIP arthritis that may be associated with PFT.

in early active finger motion. After irrigation has been completed, the distal incision is left open and the proximal incision is either left open or very loosely closed. Sometimes 5 mm of skin around the proximal incision is excised to avoid early skin closure. A soft dressing is applied, and twice a day soaks in soapy water with range of motion are started in 6 to 12 hours. The patient is typically admitted for 24 hours for intravenous antibiotics and for the first 2 to 3 soaks with the help of nursing staff. On discharge, culture-driven oral antibiotics for 10 to 14 days are given and continued twice-daily soaks with early active and passive range of motion are encouraged. If culture results have not returned by the time of patient discharge, antibiotics for a presumptive MRSA infection are given and can be changed when final culture results are in. Patients are followed closely in the office setting, typically for the first 3 to 5 days after surgery, to confirm clinical improvement. Occupational therapy is offered to patients who show slow improvement in range of motion and hand function.

OUTCOMES AND COMPLICATIONS

When left untreated, PFT can cause devastating and permanent loss of function and even amputation. Even with prompt treatment, several complications have been reported. Stern and colleagues[29] reviewed the outcome of hand infections and reported a complication rate of 38% when infection was found in the flexor tendon sheath. Stiffness, persistent infection, boutonniere deformity, and amputation were the most common complications noted in all hand infections reviewed. Pang and colleagues[12] reviewed the records of all patients diagnosed with PFT at their institution over a 5-year period and identified 5 risk factors associated with poor outcomes in PFS: (1) age greater than 43 years; (2) the presence of diabetes mellitus, peripheral vascular disease, or renal failure; (3) the presence of subcutaneous purulence; (4) digital ischemia; and (5) polymicrobial infection. Notable was that 13 of 75 patients (17%) went on to amputation of the affected digit. Final range of total active motion of surviving digits varied greatly from 4% to 100% with an average of 73%.

SUMMARY

PFT is a closed-space infection that has the potential to lead to a devastating loss of finger and hand function. It can spread rapidly into the palm, distal forearm, other digits, and nearby joints. Healthy individuals may present with no signs of systemic illness and often deny any known penetrating trauma or inoculation. Early diagnosis and prompt treatment are required to preserve the digit and prevent morbidity and loss of hand function. Many treatment options have been described, although all share 2 common principles: evacuation of the infection and tailored postoperative antibiotic treatment with close monitoring to ensure clinical improvement.

DISCLOSURE

Kanu Goyal receives or has recently received research support from Acumed and Skeletal Dynamics.

REFERENCES

1. Kanavel AB. The treatment of acute suppurative tenosynovitis- discussion of technique. In: Infections of the hand. 5th edition; 1925. p. 59–70, 225-226.
2. Glass KD. Factors related to the resolution of treated hand infections. J Hand Surg 1982;7(4):388–94.
3. Doyle JR. Anatomy of the finger flexor tendon sheath and pulley system. J Hand Surg 1988;13(4):473–84.
4. Haines SC, McCann PA. The Use of a Lacrimal Probe in Closed Catheter Irrigation of Pyogenic Flexor Tenosynovitis. Tech Orthop 2019;34(2):117–8.
5. Boles SD, Schmidt CC. Pyogenic flexor tenosynovitis. Hand Clin 1998;14(4):567–78.
6. O'Malley M, Fowler J, Ilyas AM. Community-Acquired Methicillin-Resistant Staphylococcus aureus Infections of the Hand: Prevalence and Timeliness of Treatment. J Hand Surg 2009;34(3):504–8.
7. Calhoun JH, Mader J. Musculoskeletal infections. CRC Press; 2003.
8. Bingol UA, Ulucay C, Ozler T. An unusual cause of flexor tenosynovitis: Streptococcus mitis. Plast Reconstr Surg Glob Open 2014;2(12):e263.
9. Lopez CAJ, Magee CAJ, Belyea CCM, et al. Finger flexor tenosynovitis from stonefist envenomation injury. J Am Acad Orthop Surg Glob Res Rev 2019;3(5):e024.
10. Fluke EC, Carayannopoulos NL, Lindsey RW. Pyogenic flexor tenosynovitis caused by Shewanella algae. J Hand Surg 2016;41(7):e203–6.
11. Wilhelm A, Romeo N, Trevino R. A rare cause of pyogenic flexor tenosynovitis: nocardia nova. J Hand Surg 2018;43(8):778.e1-4.
12. Pang H-N, Teoh L-C, Yam A, et al. Factors affecting the prognosis of pyogenic flexor tenosynovitis. J Bone Joint Surg Am 2007;89(8):1742–8.
13. Kanavel AB. The symptoms, signs, and diagnosis of tenosynovitis and fascial-space abscesses. In: Infections of the hand. 1st edition. Philadelphia: Lea & Febiger; 1912. p. 201–28.
14. Dailiana ZH, Rigopoulos N, Varitimidis S, et al. Purulent flexor tenosynovitis: factors influencing the functional outcome. J Hand Surg Eur Vol 2008;33(3):280–5.
15. Brusalis CM, Thibaudeau S, Carrigan RB, et al. Clinical characteristics of pyogenic flexor tenosynovitis in pediatric patients. J Hand Surg 2017;42(5):388.e1-5.
16. Yi A, Kennedy C, Chia B, et al. Radiographic soft tissue thickness differentiating pyogenic flexor tenosynovitis from other finger infections. J Hand Surg 2019;44(5):394–9.
17. Prunières G, Igeta Y, Díaz JJH, et al. Ultrasound for the diagnosis of pyogenic flexor tenosynovitis. 2018. Available at: https://www.em-consulte.com/en/article/1224427. Accessed June 11, 2019.
18. Draeger RW, Bynum DK. Flexor tendon sheath infections of the hand. J Am Acad Orthop Surg 2012;20(6):373–82.
19. Chung S-R, Foo T-L. Modifications to simplify intrathecal irrigation for pyogenic flexor tenosynovitis. Hand (N Y) 2014;9(2):258–9.
20. DiPasquale AM, Krauss EM, Simpson A, et al. Cases of early infectious flexor tenosynovitis treated nonsurgically with antibiotics, immobilization, and elevation. Plast Surg 2017;25(4):272–4. https://doi.org/10.1177/2292550317731765.
21. Bolton LE, Bainbridge C. Current opinions regarding the management of pyogenic flexor tenosynovitis: a survey of Pulvertaft Hand Trauma Symposium attendees. Infection 2019;47(2):225–31.
22. Turvey BR, Weinhold PS, Draeger RW, et al. Biomechanical effects of steroid injections used to treat pyogenic flexor tenosynovitis. J Orthop Surg 2012;7:34.
23. Gutowski K, Ochoa O, Adams W. Closed-catheter irrigation is as effective as open drainage for treatment of pyogenic flexor tenosynovitis. Ann Plast Surg 2002;49(4):350–4.
24. Born TR, Wagner ER, Kakar S. Comparison of open drainage versus closed catheter irrigation for treatment of suppurative flexor tenosynovitis. Hand (N Y) 2017;12(6):579–84.
25. Draeger R, Singh B, Bynum D, et al. Corticosteroids as an adjunct to antibiotics and surgical drainage for the treatment of pyogenic flexor tenosynovitis. J Bone Jt Surg 2010;92(16):2653–62.
26. Lille S, Hayakawa T, Neumeister MW, et al. Continuous postoperative catheter irrigation is not necessary for the treatment of suppurative flexor tenosynovitis. J Hand Surg Br Eur 2000;25(3):304–7.
27. Neviaser RJ. Closed tendon sheath irrigation for pyogenic flexor tenosynovitis. J Hand Surg 1978;3(5):462–6.
28. Knackstedt R, Tyler J, Bernard S. Closed continuous irrigation with lidocaine and immediate mobilization for treatment of pyogenic tenosynovitis. Tech Hand Up Extrem Surg 2017;21(3):114–5.
29. Stern PJ, Staneck JL, McDonough JJ, et al. Established hand infections: A controlled, prospective study. J Hand Surg 1983;8(5, Part 1):553–9.

Septic Joints: Finger and Wrist

Brian Chenoweth, MD

KEYWORDS

- Septic joint • Wrist • Metacarpophalangeal • Interphalangeal • Infection

KEY POINTS

- Common presenting symptoms of septic arthritis include joint redness, swelling, and pseudoparalysis that occurs several days following a penetrating trauma.
- Patients with immune system compromise or prosthetic joints may present with more obscure complaints and examination findings.
- Diagnostic workup should be expedited and should include bloodwork and arthrocentesis.
- Imaging, including radiographs, ultrasound, computed tomography, or MRI, can be helpful tools in diagnosis.
- Prompt surgical debridement and antibiotics are required once infection is identified.
- Stiffness is the most common complication following infection with additional reported complications including arthritis, ankylosis, and amputation.

INTRODUCTION

Patients presenting with acute monoarticular swelling, redness, and pain should receive a workup for septic arthritis. Missing or undertreating this type of infection carries significant risk of morbidity. Complications such as arthrosis, arthrofibrosis, or spread of infection can be mitigated by prompt recognition and treatment. Treatment typically requires a combination of expedient surgical debridement and appropriate antibiotic coverage. Providers also must be familiar with special circumstances, such as immunocompromised patients or patients with prosthetic joints, who may present with alternative symptomatology.

PATHOPHYSIOLOGY/EPIDEMIOLOGY

Septic joint infections typically result from direct inoculation of a joint or through hematogenous seeding.[1] Specific to joints of the hand, infections are most commonly caused by traumatic penetration of the joint capsule. Hematogenous spread is less commonly observed. Events such as a human or animal bite, laceration, or crushing injuries expose the intra-articular space to the outside environment and this results in direct inoculation of the joint with bacteria. As a result of the injury, there is production of extracellular matrix proteins that aid in joint healing. These products, such as fibronectin, promote bacterial attachment and progression to infection.[2] Bacteria express receptors that are able to recognize a variety of different host proteins. *Staphylococcus aureus* for example, produces receptors specific for laminin, fibronectin, collagen, and hyaluronic acid, among others.[3] The expression of these receptors determines whether a given bacteria will have proclivity to produce infections within the confines of a joint versus other locations within the body. Once the bacteria has invaded the host membrane, it may be internalized by native cells where it can survive, proliferate, avoid immune system surveillance, and eventually cause apoptosis and spread.[4]

Once the bacteria begins rapidly proliferating, the host immune response is activated. This results in an influx in inflammatory cells including macrophages and polymorphonuclear cells. Next, there is production of cytokines, including interleukin 1-beta and interleukin-6, tumor necrosis factor alpha, and granulocyte-macrophage

University of Oklahoma, 800 Stanton L Young Boulevard, Suite 3400, Oklahoma City, OK 73003, USA
E-mail address: cheno848@gmail.com

Hand Clin 36 (2020) 331–338
https://doi.org/10.1016/j.hcl.2020.03.006

hand.theclinics.com

colony-stimulating factor, in addition to activation of the complement system.[5] Within a few days of developing an infection, the T-cell response is induced, resulting in additional cytokines, gamma interferon, interleukin-4 and interleukin-10.[6] When the host response does not clear the infection, the immune response continues with development of high levels of these destructive by-products. This results in release of matrix metalloproteinases, lysosomal enzymes, and bacterial toxins that cause host collagen degradation. In addition, a joint effusion develops that further limits blood supply and nutrients to the intraarticular cartilage cells.[2,7] This process continues despite destruction of host tissue in an effort to limit spread of the infection to other contiguous or hematogenous locations.

CLINICAL PRESENTATION

Patients presenting with an acutely swollen, warm, or painful joint should be evaluated for septic arthritis. History of injury, such as penetrating trauma from bite, splinter, or needles, should be ascertained (**Fig. 1**). Any history of joint injection or aspiration should be documented. The patient's medical history also should be screened. In a community survey of 188 patients with septic arthritis, 84% of the adult patients were found to have an underlying medical condition and 59% had history of a joint disorder.[1] This includes conditions that may mimic infection, including gout or rheumatoid arthritis, and conditions that may weaken the immune system.

Timing of symptom onset should be obtained and time to definitive treatment should be minimized as multiple case series have shown significant deleterious effects as a result of treatment delay. Delay of more than 10 days has been associated with development of osteomyelitis and amputation.[8] The specific joint in question also may provide clues to potential mechanisms of joint seeding. The distal interphalangeal (DIP) joint may be affected by inoculation from a ruptured digital mucous cyst or by spread from nearby infections, such as a felon. The proximal interphalangeal joint (PIP) joint is vulnerable during a concomitant flexor tenosynovitis infection. Metacarpophalangeal (MP) joints are most commonly affected during clenched fist injuries, although many other mechanisms have been described.[9] Examination of the patient should also include evaluation of other contiguous and noncontiguous joints. Rates as high as 20% of oligoarticular arthritis have been reported in patients presenting with a joint infection.[10] Examination of the affected joint typically shows redness, swelling, and limitations to both active and passive motion. This is a result of the immune system producing inflammatory cytokines and increased blood flow. The high intra-articular pressure forces the joint into a position of maximum potential volume, resulting in painful pseudoparalysis.[11] The swelling that occurs may also eliminate joint creases (**Fig. 2**). Systemic symptoms, including fevers or chills, may also be present.

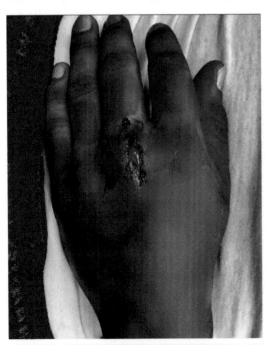

Fig. 1. This patient sustained a wound over the metacarpal phalangeal joint as a result of a closed fist injury. He presented 3 days later with redness and drainage from the wound.

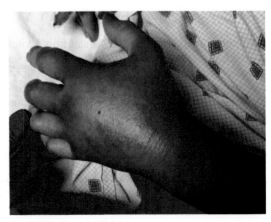

Fig. 2. Septic wrist joint.

DIAGNOSTIC WORKUP

Workup for septic arthritis typically begins with blood work including white blood cell (WBC) count with differential, C-reactive protein (CRP), and erythrocyte sedimentation rate (ESR). These tests have low specificity for septic arthritis but their sensitivity is high. Despite the high sensitivity, there have been reports of patients presenting with septic joints and normal inflammatory laboratory tests.[12] This is especially true of immunocompromised patients or patients with prosthetic joints. Another advantage of obtaining early inflammatory markers is following the trend in values during treatment to assess effectiveness. If there is any concern for systemic spread, blood cultures should be obtained as well. These cultures are ideally obtained before antibiotic administration to increase the odds of identifying the offending organism.

To differentiate septic arthritis from other causes of inflammatory arthritis, an arthrocentesis should be performed. Fluid should be sent for Gram stain and culture, and, when sufficient fluid is obtained, additional tests should be performed including WBC count with differential, atypical cultures, crystal analysis, and glucose and protein levels. A WBC count of more than 50,000/mm^3 with a polymorphonuclear count of greater than 90% has been correlated with infection in a native joint, although there is some level of overlap of those values with crystalline disease.[10] Septic arthritis can coexist with crystalline arthropathy; therefore, the presence of crystals on analysis does not rule out infection.

Imaging studies are rarely conclusive in the diagnosis of a septic arthritis case but they can provide additional information. Radiographs may show foreign bodies, fractures, chondrocalcinosis, or signs of inflammatory arthritis. Ultrasound is another modality that has a higher sensitivity for detecting effusion and can also be used to aid needle placement in the small joints of the hand and wrist. MRI may be used and is helpful to identify effusions, soft tissue abscess, and possible sites of bone involvement. Computed tomography scans have also been used to identify an effusion or abscess, although the resolution of soft tissue structures is lower when compared with MRI (**Box 1, Fig. 3**).

TREATMENT

Patients presenting with septic arthritis should be admitted for monitoring and ensuring appropriate response to treatment. If there is evidence of septic shock or organ failure, the patient should be

---

Box 1
Workup for septic joint infection

Recommended workup

- Bloodwork
  - Complete blood count with differential
  - Erythrocyte sedimentation rate
  - C reactive protein
  - Blood cultures
- Arthrocentesis
  - Gram stain and culture
  - Cell count
  - Crystal analysis
  - Protein level
  - Glucose level
- Imaging
  - Radiograph/Ultrasound/Computed tomography/MRI based on history

---

managed at an appropriate-level acute care facility.[10] Management includes a combination of prompt surgical evacuation of the infectious fluid and intravenous antibiotics. In a review of 26 patients with infection of hand joints, Sinha and colleagues[13] identified delay in onset of treatment as a predictive factor for increased postoperative stiffness. This increase in stiffness is due to the cytokines, matrix metalloproteinases, and lysosomal enzymes produced during the host immune response that combat the reproduction of the bacteria but also cause damage to host cartilage tissue. Surgical management is thus considered a surgical urgency.

Treatment options include repeated aspirations, arthroscopic drainage, and open debridement. Previous guidelines, published in 2006, report no evidence to support one treatment method versus another.[14] These guidelines, however, do not take into account the specific joint in question. Joints of the hand and wrist are notoriously more difficult to aspirate or inject than larger joints. This difficulty has been confirmed in ultrasound-based studies that confirm improved intra-articular needle positioning with image guidance.[15,16] As a result, arthrocentesis in the hand is supported more for diagnostic assistance and less for therapeutic purposes.[9] With regard to traditional arthrotomy and arthroscopic treatment of infections, a direct comparison was performed by Sammer and Shin.[17] In their series of 40 wrists, patients with a single infection site were noted to have a shorter hospital

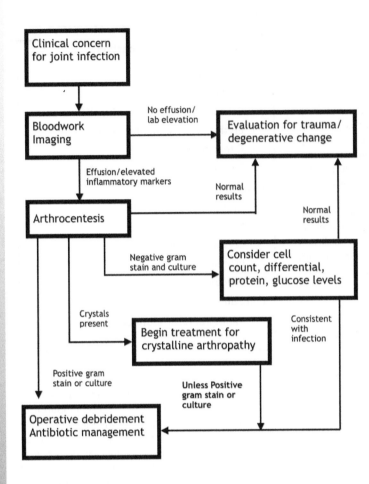

Fig. 3. Algorithm for workup of patient with acute onset of joint pain.

stay and fewer procedures when initially treated with arthroscopic drainage. These benefits were not observed in patients with multiple sites of infection.[17] No studies have been performed to date comparing open versus arthroscopic drainage in smaller joints such as the MP joint.

Arthrotomy of the wrist is typically performed through a dorsal approach. A longitudinal incision is made just ulnar to the Lister tubercle. The third compartment is opened and the extensor pollicis longus is retracted. Retinacular flaps are created to expose the fourth and fifth compartments. The posterior interosseous nerve (PIN) and its arborization into the dorsal capsule can then be identified. A neurectomy may then be performed of the PIN or it may be preserved. Neurectomy facilitates a ligament sparing approach using a radially based capsular flap, as described by Berger and Bishop.[18] A proximally based capsular flap also can be used to preserve the PIN insertion into the dorsal capsule.[19] Alternatively, capsular windows also may be created to allow access to the radiocarpal joint without creation of full capsular flaps. This exposure also allows additional

dissection to be performed to gain access to the mid carpal and distal radioulnar joint if indicated. Cultures of the joint fluid should be obtained. Infectious and nonviable tissue should then be excised and copious irrigation should be performed. The capsule may then be left open or closed over a drain based on provider preference. Similarly, skin closure may also be a loose approximation of tissue or closed over a drain.

Arthroscopic drainage begins by securing the hand into a traction tower with application of 10 to 12 pounds of traction. Gravity inflow is preferred to minimize the risk of extravasation into surrounding soft tissues. A 3 to 4 portal is created approximately 1 cm distal to the Lister tubercle. Skin only is incised with an 11-blade scalpel, followed by blunt dissection through the soft tissues with a small curved hemostat. The wrist capsule is then entered with a blunt trocar. A 6-R portal is then established between the extensor and the extensor digiti quinti and extensor carpi ulnaris. The 3 to 4 portal serves as the primary viewing portal and the 6-R serves as the primary working portal. A diagnostic arthroscopy is completed, taking note of any articular erosions or triangular fibrocartilage complex pathology. A joint shaver is then used to debride purulence and synovitis. Once this is completed, the joint is copiously irrigated with additional fluid. Once the radiocarpal joint debridement has been completed, attention may be turned to the midcarpal or distal radioulnar joint as indicated.[20]

Infections involving the MP joint are often the result of a wound that can be incorporated into the incision. A curvilinear incision is otherwise used to approach the dorsal aspect of the MP joint to avoid placing the incision directly over the extensor tendon. Dissection is performed in the subcutaneous tissues to expose and evaluate the extensor tendon for damage. An incision is made through the sagittal band to expose the joint capsule. An arthrotomy is performed and cultures are obtained of the joint fluid. The joint should then be thoroughly irrigated. Flexion should then be used to evaluate the complete surface of the metacarpal head. Injuries, such as those resulting from a clenched fist, may cause damage to the articular surface that requires debridement.[21] The capsule and sagittal band may then be left open or loosely closed followed by loose closure of the skin.

The PIP joint is typically approached through a mid-lateral approach for infection to protect the extensor mechanism. Traumatic wounds may dictate that an alternative approach, such as a dorsal approach, be used to incorporate the wound into the incision. A longitudinal incision is used and centered over the PIP joint. Careful dissection is performed to identify the lateral band. Retraction is then used to protect the lateral band dorsally and the neuromuscular bundle, which resides in the volar flap. A capsulotomy is then made through the dorsal joint capsule and accessory collateral ligament.[22] Cultures are taken of the joint fluid and then copious irrigation is performed. The articular surfaces may be inspected for erosions or to determine the extent of a trauma. Loose closure is then performed of the capsule in skin or the wound may be dressed open.

The approach to the DIP joint will typically be dictated by the inciting cause, such as a perforated digital mucous cyst or traumatic wound. An "H" style or single limb in the mid-lateral plane incision is performed. The incision can be carried distally for concomitant pathology, such as a felon. The extensor tendon is identified and carefully retracted avoiding avulsion of the tendon from the distal phalanx. An arthrotomy is then performed through the collateral ligament and dorsal capsule to expose the intraarticular space. Cultures are taken of the joint fluid and then copious irrigation is performed. The articular surfaces

may be inspected for erosions or to determine the extent of a trauma. Loose closure is then performed of the capsule in skin or the wound may be dressed open.

The patient's clinical examination and inflammatory markers should be closely monitored during the postoperative period to ensure appropriate response to therapy. If signs of infection persist, a repeat surgical debridement is performed, typically 24 to 48 hours after the index procedure. Controversy exists between early mobilization and splinting for several days to allow for soft tissue rest.[8,13,23,24] Described methods of immobilization span the spectrum of splinting for a period of days to placement of joint spanning external fixators for a period of 2 to 3 weeks. Sinha and colleagues[13] reported on 15 patients treated for metacarpophalangeal (MCP) and interphalangeal (IP) joint infections in which the patients began range of motion exercises within 24 hours. In their series, 7 patients regained full range of motion, 6 had mild stiffness, and only 3 patients had persistent pain. Another postoperative regimen involves placement of an intravenous cannula into the joint for continuous postoperative irrigation. This technique has been described for the MCP, PIP, and DIP joints.[25] Finally, some providers advocate for daily soaks in diluted solutions of povidone-iodine.[21]

Antibiotic therapy should begin immediately after obtaining the culture either by preoperative aspiration or intraoperative culture. Broad-spectrum antibiotics are initiated until culture and sensitivity results are finalized. The most commonly encountered bacteria in hand infections that should be covered by initial antibiotic choice are staphylococcal and streptococcal species, but gram-negative and anaerobic species are encountered as well.[26] Traditional antibiotic management has included several weeks of parenteral treatment followed by additional oral treatment. However, there has been increasing interest in the infectious disease literature in managing orthopedic infections with oral therapy. A large randomized control trial of more than 1000 patients was published by Li and colleagues,[27] in 2019, involving a direct comparison between parenteral versus oral treatment for complex orthopedic infections. Their results showed that treatment with oral antibiotics were noninferior with respect to treatment failure at 1 year when compared with initial treatment with 6 weeks of intravenous antibiotics. In a retrospective review of 40 adult patients specifically with hand and wrist septic joint infections, Kowalski and colleagues[26] advocated for less than 1 week of parenteral antibiotics with additional 2 to 3 weeks of oral treatment following discharge. Alternative antibiotic management would be recommended for patients with identification of mycobacterial, fungal, parasitic, or viral infections.

SPECIAL CIRCUMSTANCES

There are subgroups of patients that warrant additional discussion, including immunocompromised patients, diabetic patients, and patients with prosthetic joints. Complaints that could be consistent with infection should be carefully considered, as the chances of significant morbidity or mortality is higher in these patient populations. In a retrospective review of 110 patients with septic joints, Giuffre and colleagues[28] identified 22 infections in diabetic patients and 14 infections in patients undergoing immunosuppression therapy. They identified that the presence of diabetes and immunosuppression increased the risk of requiring an arthrodesis by 1.7 and 2.7, respectively. The risk of amputation increased by 2.1 for diabetic patients and 4.2 for patients on immunosuppression. Specific to immunosuppressed patients, in a study of 911 cardiac transplant patients, 13 infections were identified in the hand and wrist. The infections were more common in patients undergoing immunosuppression and were also frequently polymicrobial.[29] Based on the higher rate of polymicrobial infections, recommendations for antibiotic coverage includes additional coverage of fungal and anaerobic infections. Additional retrospective reviews on immunosuppressed patients have also confirmed a higher rate of amputation, longer hospital stays, and required more surgeries.[30]

Diabetic patients are at an increased risk of infection due to hyperglycemia-induced chronic neuropathy, vascular disease, and poor wound healing. Gonzalez and colleagues[31] reported on 46 upper extremity diabetic infections in which 18 patients underwent amputation and 3 deaths resulted directly from the infection. Higher chances of amputation were associated with deep infection, renal failure, and atypical/polymicrobial cultures. Jalil and colleagues[32] reported 37 diabetic hand infections with high rates of deep infection and polymicrobial growth resulting in longer hospital stays. The investigators advocated for proper glycemic control, extremity elevation, prompt surgical debridement, and appropriate antibiotics with expanded coverage.

As the use of hand and wrist arthroplasty continues to increase, upper extremity surgeons will need to become more familiar with implant-associated joint infection. In contrast to native joint infections, infections involving surgical implants involve bacterial formation of a biofilm. Bacteria bind to a physiologic film coating on the surface of the implant and develop into a bacterial colony. The colony is then able to produce an exopolymer layer that coats the colony and blocks penetration of antibiotics.[33] The formation of a colony also allows the bacteria to downregulate pathways that are typically targeted by antibiotics, making them less effective even when they penetrate the biofilm layer.[34] Once infection develops, typical signs of infection, such as fever and systemic symptoms, are often absent. Patient presentations often involve only pain and signs of radiographic loosening.[35] Additional weight is placed on the diagnostic value of arthrocentesis, as other laboratory values, including CRP and ESR, have a much lower sensitivity in prosthetic joint infections.[36] Intraoperative histopathology also may be a useful tool in determining the presence of infection. In addition to the pathogens mentioned previously, upper extremity implant-associated infections are often the result of Propionibacteria, which may require additional culture monitoring up to 14 days.

Appropriate surgical management of prosthetic joint infections is key due to limited antibiotic effectiveness. Options include debridement alone, 1-stage versus 2-stage implant replacement, explant alone, and chronic suppressive antibiotics. Debridement alone is generally reserved for acute-onset infection with a stable implant. Most infections require an implant exchange due to biofilm formation. Because the hand depends on gliding structures for function and soft tissue scarring represents significant morbidity, additional consideration is given to single-stage implant exchange. Two-stage exchange involves implant removal and temporary placement of an antibiotics cement spacer that is typically fabricated at time of surgery by the surgeon. After sufficient time has passed with appropriate antibiotic management, typically 6 to 12 weeks, the spacer is removed and a new prosthesis is placed. If the patient has poor medical status and is unable to undergo potentially multiple additional revision surgeries, consideration should be given to resection arthroplasty. If the infection is quiescent, suppressive antibiotics alone may suffice.[35]

COMPLICATIONS

The most common complication associated with infections in the joints of the hand and wrist is stiffness. In a study of 40 infections involving interphalangeal joints, only 18 patients achieved full range of motion despite a postoperative protocol, including hand therapy beginning 24 hours after surgery.[23] Another retrospective review of

26 infected joints of the hand categorized postoperative stiffness based on delay in initial treatment. Treatment delay beyond 3 days resulted in significantly higher rates of stiffness at 30% versus 77%.[13] The patient should be counseled about the potential for joint stiffness. Current evidence supports beginning range of motion exercises following surgery, although this is still controversial. Additional complications can include arthritis, ankylosis, necessity of amputation, infectious spread resulting in osteomyelitis, abscess, and ultimately mortality has been reported, although this is rare for infections of the hand. Rates of these devastating complications are greatly dependent on host factors and are more likely in patients with diabetes and on chronic immunosuppression. In a case series of 110 patients with septic interphalangeal joints, overall rates of arthrodesis and amputation were 12% and 13%, respectively, with significantly higher rates in diabetic and immunosuppressed patients.[28] Although these complications cannot be fully prevented, prompt recognition and treatment are associated with improved rates of long-term functionality.

SUMMARY

Septic joint infections in the hand and wrist carry the risk of significant morbidity if recognition and treatment are delayed. Common presenting symptoms are joint redness, swelling, and pseudoparalysis that has occurred several days following a penetrating trauma. These signs and symptoms may not be present in patients with prosthetic joints or comorbidities that compromise the immune system. Diagnostic workup should be expedited and should include laboratory evaluation and arthrocentesis. Imaging can be a helpful tool in diagnosis but is not as sensitive or specific as in other conditions. Once infection is identified, prompt surgical debridement and antibiotics are required. Previous antibiotic management has included several weeks of intravenous therapy, but recent data suggest that transitioning to oral treatment at discharge may be noninferior to a prolonged intravenous course. Once the infection has been managed, range of motion and hand therapy should be initiated to prevent stiffness, although timing in this area remains controversial.

REFERENCES

1. Kaandorp CJ, Dinant HJ, van de Laar MA, et al. Incidence and sources of native and prosthetic joint infection: a community based prospective survey. Ann Rheum Dis 1997;56(8):470–5.
2. Shirtliff ME, Mader JT. Acute septic arthritis. Clin Microbiol Rev 2002;15(4):527–44.
3. Herrmann M, Vaudaux PE, Pittet D, et al. Fibronectin, fibrinogen, and laminin act as mediators of adherence of clinical staphylococcal isolates to foreign material. J Infect Dis 1988;158(4):693–701.
4. Bayles KW, Wesson CA, Liou LE, et al. Intracellular *Staphylococcus aureus* escapes the endosome and induces apoptosis in epithelial cells. Infect Immun 1998;66(1):336–42.
5. Koch B, Lemmermeier P, Gause A, et al. Demonstration of interleukin-1beta and interleukin-6 in cells of synovial fluids by flow cytometry. Eur J Med Res 1996;1(5):244–8.
6. Abdelnour A, Bremell T, Holmdahl R, et al. Role of T lymphocytes in experimental *Staphylococcus aureus* arthritis. Scand J Immunol 1994;39(4):403–8.
7. Roy S, Bhawan J. Ultrastructure of articular cartilage in pyogenic arthritis. Arch Pathol 1975;99(1):44–7.
8. de Vries H, van der Werken C. Septic arthritis of the hand. Injury 1993;24(1):32–4.
9. Murray PM. Septic arthritis of the hand and wrist. Hand Clin 1998;14(4):579–87, viii.
10. Mathews CJ, Weston VC, Jones A, et al. Bacterial septic arthritis in adults. Lancet 2010;375(9717):846–55.
11. Horowitz DL, Katzap E, Horowitz S, et al. Approach to septic arthritis. Am Fam Physician 2011;84(6):653–60.
12. Li SF, Henderson J, Dickman E, et al. Laboratory tests in adults with monoarticular arthritis: can they rule out a septic joint? Acad Emerg Med 2004;11(3):276–80.
13. Sinha M, Jain S, Woods DA. Septic arthritis of the small joints of the hand. J Hand Surg Br 2006;31(6):665–72.
14. Weston V, Coakley G, British Society for Rheumatology (BSR) Standards, Guidelines and Audit Working Group, et al. Guideline for the management of the hot swollen joint in adults with a particular focus on septic arthritis. J Antimicrob Chemother 2006;58(3):492–3.
15. Gilliland CA, Salazar LD, Borchers JR. Ultrasound versus anatomic guidance for intra-articular and periarticular injection: a systematic review. Phys Sportsmed 2011;39(3):121–31.
16. Dubreuil M, Greger S, LaValley M, et al. Improvement in wrist pain with ultrasound-guided glucocorticoid injections: a meta-analysis of individual patient data. Semin Arthritis Rheum 2013;42(5):492–7.
17. Sammer DM, Shin AY. Comparison of arthroscopic and open treatment of septic arthritis of the wrist. J Bone Joint Surg Am 2009;91(6):1387–93.

18. Berger RA, Bishop AT, Bettinger PC. New dorsal capsulotomy for the surgical exposure of the wrist. Ann Plast Surg 1995;35(1):54–9.

19. Hagert E, Ferreres A, Garcia-Elias M. Nerve-sparing dorsal and volar approaches to the radiocarpal joint. J Hand Surg Am 2010;35(7):1070–4.

20. Sammer DM, Shin AY. Comparison of arthroscopic and open treatment of septic arthritis of the wrist. Surgical technique. J Bone Joint Surg Am 2010; 92(Suppl 1 Pt 1):107–13.

21. Wolfe SW, Scott HP, Cohen KM, et al. Green's operative hand surgery. 7th edition. Philadelphia: Elsevier; 2017. 2 volumes (xvi, 2060, I-69 pages).

22. DeDeugd CM, Rizzo M. Surgical exposure of the proximal interphalangeal joint. Hand Clin 2018; 34(2):127–38.

23. Wittels NP, Donley JM, Burkhalter WE. A functional treatment method for interphalangeal pyogenic arthritis. J Hand Surg Am 1984;9(6):894–8.

24. Mennen U, Howells CJ. Human fight-bite injuries of the hand. A study of 100 cases within 18 months. J Hand Surg Br 1991;16(4):431–5.

25. Chung SR, Kang YC, McGrouther DA. Techniques for continuous irrigation of septic joints of the hand. Tech Hand Up Extrem Surg 2019;23(3):133–7.

26. Kowalski TJ, Thompson LA, Gundrum JD. Antimicrobial management of septic arthritis of the hand and wrist. Infection 2014;42(2):379–84.

27. Li HK, Rombach I, Zambellas R, et al. Oral versus intravenous antibiotics for bone and joint infection. N Engl J Med 2019;380(5):425–36.

28. Giuffre JL, Jacobson NA, Rizzo M, et al. Pyarthrosis of the small joints of the hand resulting in arthrodesis or amputation. J Hand Surg Am 2011;36(8): 1273–81.

29. Klein MB, Chang J. Management of hand and upper-extremity infections in heart transplant recipients. Plast Reconstr Surg 2000;106(3):598–601.

30. Schmidt G, Piponov H, Chuang D, et al. Hand infections in the immunocompromised patient: an update. J Hand Surg Am 2019;44(2):144–9.

31. Gonzalez MH, Bochar S, Novotny J, et al. Upper extremity infections in patients with diabetes mellitus. J Hand Surg Am 1999;24(4):682–6.

32. Jalil A, Barlaan PI, Fung BK, et al. Hand infection in diabetic patients. Hand Surg 2011;16(3):307–12.

33. Allan RN, Skipp P, Jefferies J, et al. Pronounced metabolic changes in adaptation to biofilm growth by Streptococcus pneumoniae. PLoS One 2014; 9(9):e107015.

34. Singh R, Sahore S, Kaur P, et al. Penetration barrier contributes to bacterial biofilm-associated resistance against only select antibiotics, and exhibits genus-, strain- and antibiotic-specific differences. Pathog Dis 2016;74(6) [pii:ftw056].

35. Edwards C, Sheppard NN. Prevention, diagnosis, and treatment of implant infection in the distal upper extremity. J Hand Surg Am 2018;43(1):68–74.

36. Drago L, Vassena C, Dozio E, et al. Procalcitonin, C-reactive protein, interleukin-6, and soluble intercellular adhesion molecule-1 as markers of postoperative orthopaedic joint prosthesis infections. Int J Immunopathol Pharmacol 2011;24(2):433–40.

Necrotizing Soft Tissue Infections of the Upper Extremity

Atlee Melillo, MD, Kamal Addagatla, MD, Nicole J. Jarrett, MD*

KEYWORDS

• Necrotizing soft tissue infection • NSTI • Hand infection

KEY POINTS

• Necrotizing soft tissue infections can have varying microbiology, etiology, and risk factors for development.
• Although clinical examination is the mainstay of diagnosis, laboratory tests as well as imaging can aid in diagnosis.
• Serial surgical débridements usually are needed for treatment, with resultant defects that often require reconstruction.
• Reported rates of amputation are 22% to 37.5% and mortality from necrotizing soft tissue infections of the upper extremity is reported from 22% to 34%.
• Prompt diagnosis as well as surgical and antimicrobial treatment is necessary to decrease the risk of loss of limb or life.

INTRODUCTION

Historical evidence of necrotizing soft tissue infections (NSTIs) dates back to the fifth century BC, when Hippocrates described "erysipelas" in patients who had soft tissue infections that spread quickly and were associated with high mortality.[1] First note of such a condition in the United States was made in 1871 by the Civil War surgeon Dr Joseph Jones, who described it as "hospital gangrene."[2] These patients developed virulent, rapidly spreading infections with "grayish and greenish slough." The term "necrotizing fasciitis" later was coined by Dr B. Wilson in 1952, who noticed that the infection seemed to spare the underlying muscle yet still involved the fascial planes. This terminology was clarified further over the years, becoming known as NSTIs, in order to include cases of cellulitis and superficial skin infections because they may simply be early presentations of necrotizing fasciitis. Although no single

categorical organization for NSTIs exist, they can be separated into 4 types as follows: type I—polymicrobial/synergistic, type II—monomicrobial gram-positive (group A streptococci or *Staphylococcus aureus*), type III—monomicrobial gram-negative (typically marine-related organisms, such as *Vibrio vulnificus*), and type IV—fungal.[3] Type I is the most common accounting for 80% of the cases, followed by type II, which accounts for 10% to 15%.[4] The Centers for Disease Control and Prevention has established the Active Bacterial Core surveillance program in the United States, which reports the annual incidence of group A streptococci infections associated with either NSTI or streptococcal toxic shock syndrome. The reported incidence in 2017 was 7.26 cases per 100,000 people, leading to 0.61 deaths annually.[5] Retrospective studies from single institutions report mortality rates of 24% to 34% in confirmed cases of NSTI.[6–8] The most common site of NSTIs is the lower extremity, followed by the abdomen

Division of Plastic Surgery, Cooper University Health Care, 3 Cooper Plaza, Suite 411, Camden, NJ 08103, USA
* Corresponding author.
E-mail address: njarrett@gmail.com

Hand Clin 36 (2020) 339–344
https://doi.org/10.1016/j.hcl.2020.03.007
0749-0712/20/© 2020 Elsevier Inc. All rights reserved.

and perineum.[7] Although NSTIs of the upper extremity are less common, these infections are believed to be under-reported and are at risk of becoming more prevalent secondary to increasing intravenous drug use. This article reviews the current literature regarding clinical presentation, diagnosis, and management of NSTIs of the upper extremity.

CLINICAL PRESENTATION

A detailed patient history and focused physical examination of the upper extremity can many times alone dictate further management of NSTIs. Although any localized disruption of skin integrity can catalyze an infection, physiologic and behavioral characteristics put some patients at particularly high risk. Several single-institution retrospective studies and literature reviews have elucidated known risk factors for this condition.[6–11] Behavioral history of intravenous drug use, alcohol abuse, or cigarette smoking increases the risk of development. History of trauma, preexisting ulcers, and postoperative infection also increases the risk of development; however, one study notes a majority of case origins are unknown.[12] The most significant predictor for the development of NSTIs is a history of diabetes mellitus, as evidenced in several articles that detail patient demographics and increased risk.[6–13] Immunocompromised patients, such as those with cirrhosis, malignancy, or chronic renal failure or who are on chronic corticosteroid therapy, also are at higher risk.[9] Several studies assessing NSTIs in the upper and lower extremities identify risk factors that increase the risk of both limb loss and mortality.[10–13] A retrospective review of 1507 patients by Khamnuan and colleagues[13] showed that patients with NSTI and a history of diabetes mellitus were 3 times more likely to require an amputation involving the upper extremity, whereas chronic renal disease conferred a 2-fold risk. Another retrospective review by Chang and colleagues[11] additionally showed that peripheral vascular disease alone tripled the risk of mortality after amputation if performed more than 3 days after admission.

Traditional physical examination findings associated with NSTIs of the upper extremity include significant and rapidly spreading edema, fever, tenderness to palpation, serous or hemorrhagic bullae, skin necrosis, and foul-smelling dishwater drainage. Erythema, tenderness, and fever were found in 60% to 100% of patients in several studies.[8,9,12,14] These findings usually are apparent 12 hours to 48 hours after inoculation and can be enough to make a diagnosis. Differentiating between soft tissue cellulitis and NSTI in an early stage can be challenging, and studies have shown that the most common misdiagnosis for patients with NSTI is cellulitis.[14] Specific findings on clinical examination are known to increase the risk of amputation and mortality in patients with upper and lower extremity NSTIs. Hemorrhagic bullae seen on initial presentation is associated with approximately 5 times the risk of amputation and mortality.[11] Skin necrosis is associated with 3 times the risk of amputation and gangrene is associated with 5 times the risk.[10] **Fig. 1**A shows an example of a 65-year-old man with a history of cirrhosis who presented a few days after shucking crabs with significant edema, pain out of proportion to examination, hemorrhagic bullae, and ecchymosis. Cultures demonstrated *Vibrio vulnificus*, a type III infection.

DIAGNOSIS

Previous literature has shown that prompt diagnosis and urgent operative intervention in patients with NSTI improve outcomes. Early NSTIs can be difficult to appreciate, however, based on physical examination alone. Wong and colleagues[15] developed the Laboratory Risk Indicator for Necrotizing Fasciitis (LRINEC) score to assist in the diagnosis of clinical, early-stage NSTIs (**Table 1**). The LRINEC score is based on the following laboratory values: C-reactive protein, white blood cells,

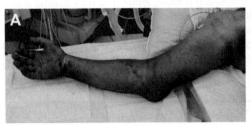 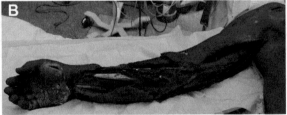

Fig. 1. A 65-year-old man with a history of cirrhosis presented a few days after shucking crabs with significant edema, pain out of proportion to examination, hemorrhagic bullae, and ecchymosis. Cultures demonstrated *Vibrio vulnificus*. Right upper extremity (*A*) on presentation and (*B*) after 2 débridements.

Table 1
Laboratory risk indicator for necrotizing fasciitis score

Variable (Units)	Score
C-reactive protein (mg/L)	
<150	0
≥150	4
Total white blood cell count (per mm³)	
<15	0
15–25	0.5
>25	2.1
Hemoglobin (g/dL)	
>13.5	0
11–13.5	0.6
<11	1.8
Sodium (mmol/L)	
≥135	0
<135	1.8
Creatinine (μmol/L)	
≤141	0
>141	1.8
Glucose (mmol/L)	
≤10	0
>10	1.2
	Total Score
Clinical suspicion for NSTI	≥6
Highly predictive of NSTI	≥8

Data from Wong CH, Khin LW, Heng KS, et al. The LRINEC (Laboratory Risk Indicator for Necrotizing Fasciitis) score: a tool for distinguishing necrotizing fasciitis from other soft tissue infections. Crit Care Med 2004;32:1535-41.

hemoglobin, sodium, creatinine, and glucose. A maximum score of at least 6 should raise clinical suspicion for NSTI, and a score of 8 or higher is strongly predictive of the disease. A meta-analysis performed in 2017 assessing the validity of the LRINEC score by Bechar and colleagues[16] noted that the average LRINEC score of 6.0 for patients with NSTI of the extremities was lower than those with NSTI of the groin (6.8) and chest/trunk (7.3). These data suggest that clinical cases of NSTIs involving the extremities have a more subtle presentation and delayed onset of sepsis. Another study assessing the reliability of the LRINEC score by Abdullah and colleagues[17] notes a sensitivity of 43.2% to 80%, a positive predictive value (PPV) of 57% to 64% and a negative predictive value (NPV) of 42% to 86%. This study concludes that the LRINEC score is reliable, and scores greater than 6 correlate with a diagnosis of NSTI (with scores >7.1 significant). Although developed as an aid to differentiate early NSTI from cellulitis, the LRINEC score

has been shown to instead confirm severe cases and predict high-risk patients with poorer outcomes.

Yoon and colleagues[18] combines the use of the LRINEC score with 2 magnetic resonance imaging (MRI) findings (intermuscular deep fascia thickening >3 mm and multicompartment involvement in 1 extremity) to differentiate NSTIs from non-NSTIs. By combining MRI findings with the LRINEC score, this study demonstrated improved sensitivity, PPV and NPV. The use of imaging studies to diagnose NSTIs, however, remains controversial. Clinical history and physical examination findings should be sufficient for diagnosis and immediate surgical débridement. Imaging can aid in diagnosis for early cases with ambiguous physical examination findings in the stable patient. Plain radiographs are of little value and are not specific enough to elucidate soft tissue gas.[19] Computed tomography (CT) scan findings include adipose tissue infiltration with edema and thickening of fascial planes, most importantly with involvement of deep fascia.[20] Edema associated with NSTI is more localized to the deeper tissues and is unevenly distributed within these fascial planes. Intravenous contrast administration is usually not necessary and can worsen acute kidney injury that often is seen in these patients. A study by McGillicuddy and colleagues[21] noted a set of CT findings that aid in the diagnosis of NSTIs that includes fascial air, muscle/fascial edema, fluid tracking, lymphadenopathy, and subcutaneous edema (**Table 2**). Points were assigned to each of these features, and a total score greater than 6 was associated with 86.3% sensitivity, 91.5% specificity, 63.3% PPV, and 85.5% NPV. The average scores for true NSTIs versus non-NSTIs were 8.57 and 2.74, respectively. The investigators note that a CT may be most useful in cases of moderate likelihood of NSTIs rather than high or low likelihood. Although literature exists detailing MRI findings sensitive and specific to NSTIs, MRI scans take a considerable time to obtain and result in further treatment delay.[20] Ultrasound imaging is a bedside tool that is less expensive and more readily available throughout the world. Castleberg and colleagues[22] describe a case report that details their use of an ultrasound to aid in the diagnosis of NSTIs by evaluating for subcutaneous thickening, air, and fascial fluid. There is no perfect imaging modality, however, that has been validated to date that can be used to diagnose NSTIs.

MEDICAL MANAGEMENT

Because patients inflicted with NSTI often can present in a state of sepsis or septic shock, it is crucial

Table 2
Characteristics of necrotizing soft tissue infections on computed tomography scan

Finding on Computed Tomography Scan	Score
Fascial air	5
Muscle/fascial edema	4
Fluid tracking	3
Lymphadenopathy	2
Subcutaneous edema	1
	Total Score
Clinical suspicion for NSTI	≥6

Data from McGillicuddy EA, Lischuk AW, Schuster KM, et al. Development of a computed tomography-based scoring system for necrotizing soft-tissue infections. J Trauma 2011;70:894-9.

to initiate appropriate resuscitation with crystalloids along with broad-spectrum antibiotics.[23] Antibiotic choice is based on known pathogens associated with the development of such infections. One study by Elliott and colleagues[24] assessing 198 patients from a single institution noted an average of 4.5 microorganisms per infection, with 98 cultures growing 4 or more pathogens. For the few cases in which 1 microorganism was isolated, that organism was usually group A streptococcus. Other common pathogens included Bacteroides, *Escherichia coli*, Enterococcus, and Staphylococcus. These findings are echoed in other microbiology studies as well.[12,23] Most patients received an average of 12.8 days of antibiotic therapy.

There are several key points to consider when selecting appropriate antibiotic coverage for treatment of NSTIs. Coverage should be broad enough to cover gram-positive, gram-negative, and anaerobic organisms. Use of vancomycin, daptomycin, or linezolid to cover methicillin-resistant staphylococcal infections until cultures have resulted also is critical. In addition, clindamycin's mechanism of action inhibits protein synthesis, resulting in decreased toxin production, particularly in infections by Streptococcus or Clostridium.[25] Recent guidelines from the Infectious Diseases Society of America suggest vancomycin or linezolid, with the addition of piperacillin-tazobactam, ceftriaxone-metronidazole, or a carbapenem.[26] Concurrent therapy for these virulent infections involves careful monitoring, usually in an intensive care unit and expectant management of multisystem organ failure. Although used almost routinely in certain centers, hyperbaric oxygen therapy still has not been scientifically proved to minimize

tissue loss and rate of amputations.[27] Intravenous immunoglobulin therapy also has been used in this setting but lacks compelling evidence for routine use.[26]

SURGICAL MANAGEMENT

Surgical management of NSTIs of the extremities is unique, given the particular importance to preserve motor and sensory functions. Although a surgeon is always trying to avoid long-term sequelae of a débridement, in cases of NSTIs, being overly conservative can result in the loss of more tissue in the future. Often, serial débridements with close monitoring for progression of infection is necessary to balance the functional and infectious concerns. A systematic review of NSTIs in the extremities from Angoules and colleagues,[9] which included 451 patients from 12 studies, noted an average of 3 surgical débridements per patient, with a range from 1 to 21 débridements. Almost half of the patients (48.8%) undergoing débridement of the upper extremity had their wounds treated with skin grafting, and 4.5% underwent rotational flap coverage. Tang and colleagues[28] published a case series for NSTIs of the upper limb that included 12 patients, with an average of 3.7 operations per patient. They suggest criteria for consideration for amputation, which include high anesthesia risk secondary to comorbidities (especially poorly controlled diabetes mellitus), necrotic underlying muscles, extensive infection or rapidly spreading infection with a large area of necrosis, septic shock requiring ionotropic support, and concurrent vascular insufficiency. With these criteria, there were 5 amputations performed, ranging from digital amputation to shoulder disarticulation. Both patients who underwent shoulder disarticulation did not survive. Case reports vary in their descriptions of surgical débridement versus amputation and wound closure.[29-31] A report by Reichert and colleagues[29] describes performing upper arm and forearm fasciotomies that required further débridement, followed by a pedicled, fasciocutaneous parascapular flap and a free ipsilateral anterolateral thigh flap for ultimate closure of these wounds. A report by Hankins and Southern[30] describes a case involving 6 surgical operations over the course of 9 hospital days to control an infection. These procedures included several sessions of irrigation and débridement along with resection of the extensor tendon of the left middle finger. The wound was dressed temporarily with a silicone/nylon skin substitute. The final reconstructive surgery consisted of an anterior lateral thigh flap to the dorsum of the hand and a silastic rod to replace his previous tendon in a staged fashion. A case report by Minini and colleagues[31] details an extensive infection from the dorsum of the hand to the distal forearm. The case was treated with 3 surgeries, culminating in an amputation of the third ray, wedge osteotomy of the capitate, closure of the metacarpal space with cerclages, and a fasciocutaneous posterior interosseous flap. **Fig. 1**B demonstrates an example of the patient, discussed previously, with an NSTI of the upper extremity after débridement. Unfortunately, the amount of infected and necrotic tissue was so profound that despite prompt surgical and medical management, the patient succumbed to multisystem organ failure.

Surgical management for NSTIs of the upper extremity is case specific and largely depends on the hemodynamic status of the patient and the extent of disease. Patients and their families must be informed of the need for serial surgeries and possibly complex reconstructions in the future.

OUTCOMES

Few studies report functional outcomes of infections associated with the hand and are limited to case studies.[30–32] Rates of amputation for NSTIs of the upper extremity range from 22% to 37.5%.[28,32] Increased amputation rate has been associated with sepsis and history of diabetes.[32] Avoidance of amputation has been associated with early diagnosis and prompt treatment with antibiotics and operative débridement.[7,9,10] Data on wound closure and dressing choice usually are limited to case reports, but one study details the use of negative-pressure wound therapy with no discernible impact on patient outcome.[33] The decision to amputate should be unique to an individual case and rely on the extent of infection and hemodynamic status of the patient. Reported mortality rates for NSTIs of the upper extremity range from 22% to 34%.[10,28] Increased mortality is associated with increased age, liver dysfunction, and proximal extent of infection on the limb.[32]

SUMMARY

Although literature is still sparse on NSTIs specific to the upper extremity, it is clear that this subset of cases presents a unique challenge to the surgeon. Prompt diagnosis and early operative intervention are critical in managing these patients. Although extra caution is necessary in these cases to preserve upper extremity function, NSTIs of the upper extremity often can have delayed onset of true severity. Therefore, upfront aggressive management is recommended to preserve life over limb.

DISCLOSURE

There are no commercial or financial conflicts of interest from any of the authors.

REFERENCES

1. Descamps V, Aitken J, Lee MG. Hippocrates on necrotizing fasciitis. Lancet 1994;344:556.
2. Jones J. Observations upon the losses of the Confederate armies from battle, wounds and disease during the American Civil War of 1861–1865, with investigations upon the number and character of the diseases supervening upon gun-shot wounds. The Richmond and Louisville Med J 1869;8:340–58.
3. Morgan MS. Diagnosis and management of necrotizing fasciitis: a multiparametric approach. J Hosp Infect 2010;75:249–57.
4. Mishra SP, Singh S, Gupta SK. Necrotizing soft tissue infections: surgeon's prospective. Int J Inflam 2013;2013:609–28.
5. Centers for Disease Control and Prevention. 2017. Active bacterial core surveillance report, emerging infections program network, Group A Streptococcus 2017. Available at: http://www.cdc.gov/abcs/reports-findings/survreports/gas17.pdf.
6. Anaya DA, McMahon K, Nathens AB, et al. Predictors of mortality and limb loss in necrotizing soft tissue infections. Arch Surg 2005;140:151–7.
7. Cheung JP, Fung B, Tang WM, et al. A review of necrotising fasciitis in the extremities. Hong Kong Med J 2009;15:44–52.
8. Zhao JC, Zhang BR, Shi K, et al. Necrotizing soft tissue infection: clinical characteristics and outcomes at a reconstructive center in Jilin Province. BMC Infect Dis 2017;171:792.
9. Angoules AG, Kontakis G, Drakoulakis E, et al. Necrotising fasciitis of upper and lower limb: a systematic review. Injury 2007;38:S19–26.
10. Ozalay M, Ozkoc G, Akpinar S, et al. Necrotizing soft-tissue infection of a limb: clinical presentation and factors related to mortality. Foot Ankle Int 2006;27:598–605.
11. Chang CP, Hsiao CT, Lin CN, et al. Risk factors for mortality in the late amputation of necrotizing fasciitis: a retrospective study. World J Emerg Surg 2018;13:45.
12. Wong CH, Chang HC, Pasupathy S, et al. Necrotizing fasciitis: clinical presentation, microbiology, and determinants of mortality. J Bone Joint Surg Am 2003;85:1454–60.
13. Khamnuan P, Chongruksut W, Jearwattanakanok K, et al. Necrotizing fasciitis: epidemiology and clinical predictors for amputation. Int J Gen Med 2015;8:195–202.
14. Singh G, Bharpoda P, Reddy R. Necrotizing Fasciitis: A Study of 48 Cases. Indian J Surg 2015;77:345–50.

15. Wong CH, Khin LW, Heng KS, et al. The LRINEC (Laboratory Risk Indicator for Necrotizing Fasciitis) score: a tool for distinguishing necrotizing fasciitis from other soft tissue infections. Crit Care Med 2004;32:1535–41.

16. Bechar J, Sepehripour S, Hardwicke J, et al. Laboratory risk indicator for necrotising fasciitis (LRINEC) score for the assessment of early necrotising fasciitis: a systematic review of the literature. Ann R Coll Surg Engl 2017;99:341–6.

17. Abdullah M, McWilliams B, Khan SU. Reliability of the Laboratory Risk Indicator in Necrotising Fasciitis (LRINEC) score. Surgeon 2019;17(5):309–18.

18. Yoon MA, Chung HW, Yeo Y, et al. Distinguishing necrotizing from non-necrotizing fasciitis: a new predictive scoring integrating MRI in the LRINEC score. Eur Radiol 2019;29:3414–23.

19. Fugitt JB, Puckett ML, Quigley MM, et al. Necrotizing fasciitis. Radiographics 2004;24:1472–6.

20. Malghem J, Lecouvet FE, Omoumi P, et al. Necrotizing fasciitis: contribution and limitations of diagnostic imaging. Joint Bone Spine 2013;80:146–54.

21. McGillicuddy EA, Lischuk AW, Schuster KM, et al. Development of a computed tomography-based scoring system for necrotizing soft-tissue infections. J Trauma 2011;70:894–9.

22. Castleberg E, Jenson N, Dinh VA. Diagnosis of necrotizing faciitis with bedside ultrasound: the STAFF Exam. West J Emerg Med 2014;15:111–3.

23. Anaya DA, Dellinger EP. Necrotizing soft-tissue infection: diagnosis and management. Clin Infect Dis 2007;44:705–10.

24. Elliott D, Kufera JA, Myers RA. The microbiology of necrotizing soft tissue infections. Am J Surg 2000; 179:361–6.

25. Stevens DL, Bryant AE, Hackett SP. Antibiotic effects on bacterial viability, toxin production, and host response. Clin Infect Dis 1995;20:S154–7.

26. Stevens DL, Bryant AE. Necrotizing Soft-Tissue Infections. N Engl J Med 2017;377:2253–65.

27. Levett D, Bennett MH, Millar I. Adjunctive hyperbaric oxygen for necrotizing fasciitis. Cochrane Database Syst Rev 2015;(1):CD007937.

28. Tang WM, Ho PL, Fung KK, et al. Necrotising fasciitis of a limb. J Bone Joint Surg Br 2001;83:709–14.

29. Reichert JC, Habild G, Simon P, et al. Necrotizing streptococcal myositis of the upper extremity: a case report. BMC Res Notes 2017;10:407.

30. Hankins CL, Southern S. Factors that affect the clinical course of group A beta- haemolytic streptococcal infections of the hand and upper extremity: a retrospective study. Scand J Plast Reconstr Surg Hand Surg 2008;42:153–7.

31. Minini A, Galli S, Salvi AG, et al. Necrotizing fasciitis of the hand: a case report. Acta Biomed 2018;90: 162–8.

32. Nazerani S, Maghari A, Kalantar Motamedi MH, et al. Necrotizing fasciitis of the upper extremity, case report and review of the literature. Trauma Mon 2012;17:309–12.

33. Corona PS, Erimeiku F, Reverte-Vinaixa MM, et al. Necrotising fasciitis of the extremities: implementation of new management technologies. Injury 2016; 47(Suppl 3):S66–71.

Hand Infections Associated with Systemic Conditions

Zachary J. Finley, MD, Gleb Medvedev, MD*

KEYWORDS

• Hand • Infection • HIV • Diabetes • Rheumatoid • Systemic disease • Systemic conditions

KEY POINTS

- Human immunodeficiency virus–positive patients are at increased risk for atypical hand infections, including viral and fungal pathogens.
- Diabetics are at increased risk for hand infections associated with severe complications, including necrotizing fasciitis.
- Patients on immunosuppressive therapy, including those who are posttransplant or on disease-modifying antirheumatic drugs for autoimmune disorders, are at increased risk for deep structure hand infections.
- Immunocompromised patients require broad spectrum antibiotic and antifungal coverage as well as early aggressive surgical intervention in cases of necrotizing soft tissue infection.

INTRODUCTION

Life expectancies for many systemic conditions, including human immunodeficiency virus (HIV), diabetes mellitus (DM), and rheumatoid arthritis (RA), have increased with more effective treatment regimens available. Such patients are at higher risk for infection because of their immunocompromised state. The higher incidence of complications due to upper extremity infections is well established for these patients. More specifically, treating physicians are increasingly encountering hand infections and, therefore, the management of these infections in patients with systemic conditions has become increasingly relevant. Furthermore, approaches to management of hand infections require individualized care and special consideration to the patient's healing potential within the context of the specific systemic condition. In this article, the authors aim to provide an overview of the presentation of hand infections in patients with associated systemic conditions and a review of the most current methods, techniques, evidence, and controversies in the management and treatment of hand infections for patients with HIV and diabetes mellitus; approaches for infection management in the setting of RA, tuberculosis, and transplant patients are also briefly discussed.

OVERVIEW

Systemic conditions such as HIV, diabetes mellitus, and RA place patients at higher risk for hand infections for various reasons. This risk is also shared by patients on immunosuppressive therapies. At-risk patients commonly present atypically due to increased susceptibility to a broader spectrum of causative organisms including viruses, fungi, and rare bacteria. Compromised immune systems and delayed recognition of symptoms further increase the risk to these patients for deeper and more severe infections, including necrotizing fasciitis. A high level of clinical

Department of Orthopaedic Surgery, Tulane University School of Medicine, 1430 Tulane Avenue, New Orleans, LA 70112, USA
* Corresponding author.
E-mail address: gmedvede@tulane.edu

Hand Clin 36 (2020) 345–353
https://doi.org/10.1016/j.hcl.2020.03.008
0749-0712/20/© 2020 Elsevier Inc. All rights reserved.

hand.theclinics.com

suspicion by the treating physician and a well-rounded knowledge base, coupled with the use of aggressive, broad spectrum therapies, lead to improved outcomes. Further research will clarify the efficacy of specific antibiotic and antifungal regimens and the optimal perioperative timing for immunosuppressive pharmacologic agents.

HUMAN IMMUNODEFICIENCY VIRUS

HIV compromises the immune system through the destruction of CD4 cells, which are responsible for fighting infection as part of the adaptive immune system of the host. Although this diagnosis was commonly a death sentence in decades past, improvements in treatment have significantly decreased mortality for HIV patients and consequently, have increased the prevalence of the disease in the population. HIV treatments have primarily focused on decreasing the viral load, leading to higher CD4 cell counts. Although life expectancies have increased secondary to improved treatments, patients with HIV remain at a higher risk for developing hand infections. Unlike hand infections resulting from trauma as found in the general population, infections in HIV patients are more likely to be spontaneous.[1] In addition, HIV-positive patients require increased lengths of hospital stay, especially for those with decreased CD4 counts.[2]

Diagnosis/Presentation

Certain social behaviors that place these patients at higher risk for contracting systemic disease, such as increased incidence of intravenous drug use and risky sexual behavior, also place them at higher risk for contracting infections of the hand and upper extremity. In a study by Gonzalez and colleagues,[3] investigators found that of 28 infections involving the upper extremity in HIV-positive patients, 16 of them developed after intravenous injection of illicit drugs. Seven of the infections were developed at the site of a laceration or other injury. As with other infections, common symptoms include pain, swelling, or discoloration to a portion of the hand, for a prolonged length of time. Episodes of drainage or foul smell should be ascertained. A thorough medical history is critical given the common complexity of medical problems.

Treatment

Much of the presentation and treatment of these infections depends on the causative organism. Staphylococcus aureus (S aureus) is the most common cause of infection in HIV-positive individuals.[4] Other common organisms include alpha hemolytic streptococcus and beta hemolytic streptococcus. An abscess is the most common presentation for a hand infection in an HIV-positive patient due to one of these common bacterial infections.[3] Treatment can differ in timing and duration. The clinical course of the infection is often more severe and requires more prompt and aggressive treatment, even for those HIV patients whose presentation is similar to patients without HIV.

In the setting of an abscess or suspicion of necrotizing fasciitis, urgent or emergent surgical intervention is necessary. Most HIV-positive patients presenting with abscesses involving the hand should be treated with incision and drainage. One-time incision and drainage, in combination with intravenous antibiotics, has been shown to be an effective treatment in these cases with abscess formation secondary to bacterial infection.[3] A broader spectrum of antibiotics is required to cover atypical pathogens associated with HIV. In addition, duration of antibiotics tends to be extended in these patients.

In addition to common bacterial infections of the hand, HIV-positive patients are at an increased risk for viral and fungal infections that are less commonly seen in everyday practice. Examples of these include herpes simplex virus (HSV), human papillomavirus (HPV), and opportunistic fungal infections including Candida albicans and Cryptococcus.

Incision and drainage should be avoided in abscess formation secondary to viral or fungal infection, as this can lead to secondary bacterial infection. Viral or fungal infection can sometimes mimic bacterial abscess formation and should therefore be ruled out.

Herpetic Whitlow

Herpetic whitlow is a viral infection of the hand caused by HSV-1 and -2. Herpetic whitlow has a higher prevalence in HIV-positive patients and has even been reported to be the first manifestation of previously undiagnosed HIV.[5] Presentation classically begins with a single vesicle or cluster of vesicles that arise on a single-digit days after minor trauma to the skin. Most frequent locations include the terminal phalanx of the thumb, index, or long finger near the nail. These vesicles will then coalesce to form a larger bulla, similar in appearance to a bacterial felon or paronychia, with symptoms including pain, erythema, and swelling (**Fig. 1**). Notable distinctions include formation of nonpurulent vesicles or bullae, as well as maintenance of the tension in the pulp space of the digit, which is not increased unless secondary bacterial infection is present. Laboratory

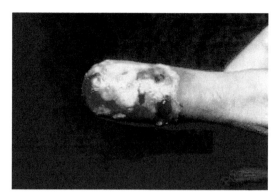

Fig. 1. Herpetic whitlow. (*Courtesy of* P.A. Volberding, MD, San Francisco, CA.)

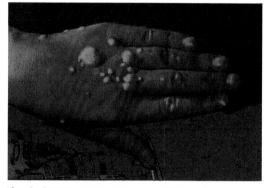

Fig. 2. Severe cutaneous warts (HPV infection) in a boy with HIV infection. (*Courtesy of* Pediatric AIDS Pictorial Atlas, Baylor International Pediatric AIDS Initiative, Texas Children's Hospital, Houston, TX.)

diagnosis involves Tzanck smear of scrapings, serum antibody titers, lesion-specific antigen detection, and viral cultures.[6]

Often thought to be interchangeable, the terms "whitlow" and "felon" in the context of herpetic whitlow are distinct conditions. The more general term "felon" is not representative of the presentation or the treatment of herpetic whitlow. This misnomer is especially controversial because it relates to treatment. Although bacterial whitlows require incision and drainage, incision and drainage in HSV infection is contraindicated because it can potentially lead to secondary bacterial infection.[7] The natural history of herpetic whitlow is complete resolution within 3 weeks; therefore, usual treatment is limited to observation to ensure secondary bacterial infection does not occur. However, for HIV and other immunocompromised patients, additional treatment is often required in the form of oral or intravenous acyclovir, valacyclovir, famciclovir, or foscarnet.[6]

Human Papillomavirus

HPV is the virus responsible for causing warts of the hand. Presentation of these warts involves raised, demarcated, grayish lesions with an irregular surface, occurring anywhere on the hand (**Fig. 2**). They are often described as having a cauliflower appearance and historically have been a condition associated with poultry and meat handlers.[6] Today, however, the more common presentation may perhaps be in the immunocompromised patient. Typically, the course of HPV is self-limited in the immunocompetent patient with warts primarily affecting cosmesis; however, in the HIV population they often persist and spread. Warts can be bothersome if their location is at a pressure point during grip or in the periungual area where they can extend into the nail bed and

under the nail plate, potentially causing destruction to the distal phalanx.[6]

Treatment of hand warts in HIV patients typically begins nonsurgically, including freezing with liquid nitrogen, electrodiathermy, or acid preparations. Recurrence rates with conservative treatments are relatively high in this population.[8] If more conservative treatments fail, surgical excision is indicated to prevent spread and continued irritation. HPV has also been identified as a causative factor for invasive squamous cell carcinoma of the nail bed in patients with AIDS, necessitating varying levels of amputation.[9] Milder forms of squamous cell carcinoma, specifically Bowen disease of the hand, a form of squamous cell carcinoma in situ, have also been linked to chronic HPV infection, with immunosuppression playing an important role in the pathogenesis of Bowen disease.[10]

Fungal Infections

HIV increases susceptibility to fungal infections of the hand, most commonly *Cryptococcus* and *C albicans*. *C albicans* typically presents with onycholysis and tends to display a more chronic course in the setting of HIV as opposed to immunocompetent patients (**Fig. 3**).[1] Although topical antifungals can be used, the most common of which include ciclopirox, amorolfine, tioconazole, and terbinafine gel, topical agents alone have a low cure rate. Therefore, they are often used in conjunction with a systemic oral agent or in severe cases after surgical removal of the nail.[6] Systemic oral agents include terbinafine and itraconazole.[11] *Cryptococcus* is an opportunistic infectious fungus that disproportionately affects patients with AIDS. In this population it has been found to cause skin lesions, tenosynovitis, and even necrotizing fasciitis.[8] Diagnosis is made via tissue biopsy

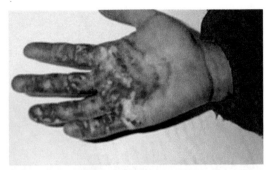

Fig. 3. Candidiasis of the hand. (*Courtesy of* Pediatric AIDS Pictorial Atlas, Baylor International Pediatric AIDS Initiative, Texas Children's Hospital, Houston, TX.)

and culture, which characteristically show encapsulated, ovoid yeasts. Treatment involves antifungals amphotericin B with flucytosine or fluconazole as an alternative therapy.[6]

Complications

Complications in HIV patients are often secondary to missed diagnosis. For example, herpetic whitlow has been misdiagnosed as a bacterial infection and consequently treated with incision and attempted drainage, only to result in secondary bacterial infection.[12] Complications are more prevalent in this population of patients because of the variability in their immune response to treatment. Severe complications, such as necrotizing fasciitis, have been reported; these complications can be caused by numerous organisms in this population.[1]

DIABETES MELLITUS

As with HIV, patients with diabetes mellitus are at an increased risk for hand infections. This is secondary to multifactorial predisposition. Patients with diabetes are often immunocompromised as a result of extended periods of hyperglycemia, which leads to decreased neutrophil activity and chemotaxis secondary to leukocyte adhesion. In addition, diabetic patients are predisposed to peripheral neuropathy and vascular disease, both of which compromise wound healing and lead to more severe infections at initial presentation.[1] All of these factors make hand infections in diabetics challenging to treat. Particular care and attention are needed for successful treatment.

Diagnosis/Presentation

Presentation of hand infections in diabetic patients varies. Particularly in the setting of neuropathy, presentation may be delayed, leading to more

severe infection at first presentation. Diabetes is also a known risk factor for necrotizing fasciitis, and therefore a high clinical suspicion is necessary to prevent delayed treatment in the setting of this surgical emergency.[13] Compared with nondiabetics, diabetic hand infections are more likely to present as osteomyelitis or septic arthritis.[14]

As in HIV patients, causative organisms play a critical role in diabetic hand infections. They are more likely to be polymicrobial or fungal on final culture.[14] Diabetic patients are more predisposed to fungal infections specifically because of physiologic changes associated with hyperglycemia.[14] For example, *Candida* species have increased adhesion to the epithelium because of glycosylated proteins,[15] ketone reductases create high-glucose conditions that are favorable for *Rhizopus* species,[16] and diabetes mellitus hyperglycemia impairs macrophage ability to kill *Burkholderia pseudomallei*, thereby increasing the risk of melioidosis.[17]

Treatment

Treatment of hand and upper extremity infections in diabetics pose a more complex challenge than in the nondiabetic population. They have been shown to more likely require repeat surgical drainage and eventual amputation. In a study by Sharma and colleagues,[14] 50% of diabetic hand and upper extremity infections that were initially treated with incision and drainage required repeat drainage; of these, 12% went on to amputation. In nondiabetic patients, repeat drainage rates were 24%, and amputations among this group were 3%. Because of the increased prevalence of fungal pathology as described earlier, it is important to send samples taken at the time of surgery for fungal stain and cultures, in addition to the traditional aerobic and anaerobic workup.

Another important consideration for diabetics is the variability in presentation based on glycemic control. As described previously, a hyperglycemic environment has been shown to be more favorable to infection of certain fungal species including *Candida, Rhizopus,* and *B pseudomallei*, suggesting that poorer glycemic control increases susceptibility to infection by these organisms. In addition, Sharma and colleagues[14] have shown that periinfection glycemic control in these patients affects outcomes. Patients demonstrating poor inpatient glycemic control, defined as average blood glucose of 180 mg/dL or greater during hospitalization, were significantly more likely to require repeat surgical intervention during the course of treatment. This finding suggests that tighter glycemic control during treatment of hand infections in diabetics could be beneficial. Research findings by Stepan and colleagues[18] provide further evidence in support of improved treatment response in patients with adequate glycemic control. The study found a greater risk for surgical complications, including postoperative infection, in insulin-dependent diabetics compared with nondiabetics, whereas no significant difference was found in noninsulin-dependent diabetics compared with nondiabetics in the setting of upper extremity procedures.

Necrotizing Fasciitis

Diabetes mellitus has been shown to be the most common comorbidity in the setting of necrotizing fasciitis, with a contributing role in as many as 70% of necrotizing fasciitis cases.[19] This surgical emergency is marked by rapidly progressive infection primarily involving the fascia and subcutaneous tissue with thrombosis of the cutaneous microcirculation. Other risk factors include alcohol abuse and intravenous drug use. When presenting in the upper extremity, initial infection can misleadingly seem benign, often resulting in delayed diagnosis, increased morbidity, and death.[20] Presentation is often similar in appearance to a low-grade cellulitis; clinical signs then rapidly progress to crepitus, fluctuance, nonpitting edema, diffuse pain, hypotension, fever, and tachycardia. Later findings include skin sloughing, blistering, ischemia, and skin necrosis (**Fig. 4**).[21,22] High clinical suspicion is required to avoid missing this time-sensitive diagnosis.

Treatment involves aggressive, urgent surgical debridement of involved soft tissue in addition to broad spectrum intravenous antibiotics. Wounds are typically left open following debridement, with repeat visits to the operating room for serial debridement every 24 to 48 hours as needed. Initial antibiotics should target aerobes and anaerobes; effective treatment often requires the administration of multiple drugs simultaneously. Most commonly, polymicrobial agents are the cause of infection in the diabetic population and, therefore, broad spectrum coverage is critical. Suggested combinations include ampicillin-sulbactam, clindamycin, and ciprofloxacin.[22] Aerobes, anaerobes, gram-negative, and gram-positive organisms have all been isolated from necrotizing infections, and it is thought that the synergistic action of multiple organisms can lead to the fascial necrosis and systemic toxicity associated with this infection.[23] The most common causative pathogens involved with polymicrobial necrotizing fasciitis include streptococcus and Enterobacter species. Among those cases of monomicrobial

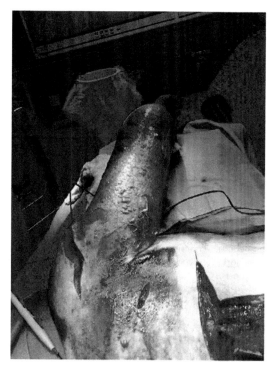

Fig. 4. Necrotizing fasciitis involving the upper extremity. (*Courtesy of* A. Ward, MD, Charlotte, NC.)

infection, Group A streptococcus has been found to be the most commonly isolated organism.[19]

Fungal infection has also been cited as a cause of necrotizing fasciitis in the hand and upper extremity in diabetic patients.[24] *Mucormycosis* is a fungal organism characteristically found in soil, plants, and decaying material. It disproportionately affects diabetic patients and is notoriously morbid, secondary to vascular thrombosis and gangrenous tissue necrosis. The most commonly implicated mucormycoses include *Mucor, Rhizopus,* and *Absidia*. If fungal infection is suspected, aggressive surgical debridement and an antifungal agent such as amphotericin B with flucytosine are indicated. Increased mortality, ranging from 23% to 76%, is significantly associated with a delay in diagnosis; surgical debridement and amputation may be necessary to control the spread of infection.[19,23]

Wounds contaminated with soil or gravel can increase risk of *Mucormycosis* infection.[25] Clinical presentation consists of enlarging black skin eschar with or without gangrene. Biopsy results characteristically show fungal organisms scattered within areas of necrosis and 90° hyphae on KOH stain (**Fig. 5**).[26] Treatment is aggressive with early, radical surgical debridement in combination with high-dose intravenous administration of amphotericin B.[6] The clinical course of fungal

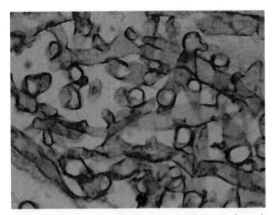

Fig. 5. Periodic acid-Schiff staining showing broad-based, ribbonlike, nonseptate hyphae with 90° branching, characteristic of *Mucormycosis*. (*From* Lass-Flörl C. Zygomycosis: conventional laboratory diagnosis. Clin Microbiol Infect 2009;15 Suppl 5:60-65; with permission.)

infection due to contaminated trauma can be particularly devastating; therefore, prompt recognition with initiation of treatment is vital in order to preserve the limb. If the infection progresses to necrotizing fasciitis, mortality rates as high as 80% have been reported.[27] In one study of 7 patients with upper extremity mucormycosis infection after traumatic injury, Moran and colleagues[28] reported an average of 10 surgical debridements for each patient, with 4 out of 7 patients ultimately requiring upper extremity amputation at varying levels ranging from fingers to glenohumeral joint disarticulation.

OTHER SYSTEMIC CONDITIONS
Rheumatoid Arthritis

Rheumatoid arthritis is an autoimmune disorder affecting 1% of the population. The small joints and soft tissues of the hand and wrist are commonly involved.[29] Effective treatments have been developed that have greatly improved the natural history of this disease including disease-modifying antirheumatic drugs (DMARDs), such as methotrexate, and steroids such as prednisolone. Newer biologics used for RA treatment include tumor necrosis factor (TNF) blockers, interleukin 1 antagonists, interleukin 6 antagonists, anti-CD28, and anti-B cell agents.[30] These pharmacologic agents effectively treat rheumatic disease and other autoimmune disorders through immunosuppression. They have been shown to substantially improve clinical and radiographic indicators when compared with traditional DMARDs, especially in patients with poor response to traditional therapies. However, it is

theorized that these newer biologics place patients at higher risk for infection in the hand and upper extremity. Data supporting this theory are inconsistent and drug dependent.

Jain and colleagues[29] studied the influence of steroids and methotrexate on wound complications after elective rheumatoid hand and wrist surgery. With the exception of diabetic patients, the study reported no statistically significant risk of wound infection or breakdown in patients treated with these medications. A systematic review and meta-analysis by Singh and colleagues[30] assessed the risk of serious infection in patients with RA treated with biologics. This study compared the risk of infection in patients undergoing traditional DMARD therapy versus newer biologics. They found that use of these newer biological agents, with or without concomitant use of DMARDs, are associated with an increased risk of serious infection in RA compared with traditional DMARDs. This held for both standard and high-dose biological drugs, whereas no increased risk was seen with low-dose biological drugs.[30]

An observational study by Berthold and colleagues[31] looked at comparative risk of surgical site infection in rheumatic patients on TNF blockade who underwent elective orthopedic and hand surgeries. They found no significant difference in rates of infection in patients undergoing elective hand surgery, whether TNF inhibitors were discontinued or maintained during the perioperative period. They did, however, find a significantly higher rate of infection in patients undergoing elective foot surgery who continued with TNF inhibitors.

Tuberculosis

Mycobacterium tuberculosis is the causative organism in tuberculosis (TB). Although uncommon, TB is still seen in immunocompromised patients. Extrapulmonary TB has been reported in the hand and can present with cutaneous infections, tenosynovitis, osteomyelitis, septic arthritis, and dactylitis.[6] Tubercles, also known as rice bodies, can grow on the walls of the tenosynovium, leading to tenosynovitis and carpal tunnel syndrome via extension into the carpal tunnel. These tubercles contain live mycobacteria that grow on culture, with pathologic specimens showing characteristic caseating granulomas.[6] TB can invade virtually any structure in the hand leading to unifocal or multifocal osteomyelitis, cystic lesions, cutaneous nodules, and hypersensitivity-type reaction with aseptic arthritis and soft tissue swelling.[32] Treatment of TB of the hand is primarily nonsurgical and involves triple therapy with isoniazid, rifampin, and pyrazinamide, with or without ethambutol, for at least 2 months. After the initial 2 months, isoniazid and rifampin are continued for an additional 4 months. Longer treatment regimens of up to 18 months have also been proposed.[6]

Transplant Patients

Transplant patients are at increased risk for hand infections secondary to immunosuppressive therapy. Similar to HIV, these patients present with increased occurrence of fungal and polymicrobial infection.[1] Klein and Chang[33] investigated the management of hand and upper-extremity infection in 911 heart transplant patients over the course of 30 years. They found 13 of these patients were treated for hand infections, with 46% found to have fungal infections and 8% with mycobacterial infections. Seventy-seven percent required operative debridement and 23% underwent more than one operative procedure. Their final recommendations involved empirical coverage for gram-positive, gram-negative, anaerobic, and fungal organisms in these patients until culture and sensitivities finalize. A study by Francel and colleagues[34] echoed the severity of infection in these patients. The study found similar severity in hand infections of diabetic patients who had undergone renal transplants. The entire transplant study group (100%) eventually required amputation compared with 51.6% in the nontransplant group.

Mull and colleagues[35] recently reported on surgical upper extremity infections in immunosuppressed patients, retrospectively comparing 2 match-paired groups. Immunosuppressive therapy included primarily glucocorticoids as well as biologics and TNF-alpha inhibitors. Patients included transplant patients and those with autoimmune disease and hematologic malignancy diagnoses. Investigators found that infections in immunosuppressed patients were more likely to involve deeper anatomy such as joints, bone, tendon sheath, muscle, or fascia and were less likely to present with leukocytosis. In addition, immunosuppressed patients more commonly exhibited atypical organisms such as *mycoplasma* or fungi. They found no difference between the groups in terms of length of hospital stay or need for repeat surgical drainage. The investigators concluded that the mechanism and white blood cell count are less reliable markers for infection severity in immunosuppressed patients compared with noncompromised patients.

SUMMARY

Much of the research regarding hand infections in HIV patients is now decades old. Further studies are needed to understand how these infections present and how approaches to management have changed, given the marked improvement in patient outcomes as a result of newer systemic treatments of HIV. Nevertheless, HIV patients across the spectrum of the disease continue to present, and a well-rounded understanding of the natural course of the condition is necessary. Hand infection may be the first manifestation of HIV in a patient, making the hand surgeon the first provider to see and recognize these patients.[5]

Hand infections in the setting of diabetes presents a complex problem, given the increased risk of polymicrobial infection, the prevalence of associated systemic conditions, and the high-risk rapid progression of severe infection. This can be secondary to delayed presentation because of neuropathy or causative organisms leading to necrotizing soft tissue infection. Close attention must be paid to these patients because of these risk factors, and aggressive early treatment is paramount. Tight glycemic control in the perioperative period may lead to decreased postoperative infection risk, and further research in this area is warranted.

The use of newer biological DMARDs for treatment of RA and their role in hand infections remain unclear. Few studies exist, and they focus on the use of these medications in the context of surgery. Guidelines for perioperative use of these agents surrounding hip and knee replacement were released in 2017 jointly by the American College of Rheumatology and American Association of Hip and Knee Surgeons.[36] Their recommendations include holding medication before surgery between 9 weeks to 2 days, based on individual medication dosing interval. Postoperatively, medication can be restarted once the incisional wound seems to be healing or around 2 weeks following surgery. Currently there is no consensus guideline for perioperative use of these medications in hand surgery.[1] Whether or not these or similar guidelines can be applied to hand surgery remains to be seen. More research is warranted to understand the mechanism of action of these newer RA medications in hand infections generally and their use in perioperative management of hand surgery.

Extrapulmonary TB has been identified as one causative agent in hand infections. Although these infections can invade virtually any structure in the hand leading to osteomyelitis, cystic lesions, cutaneous nodules, aseptic arthritis, and soft tissue swelling, treatment protocols are well established.

For immunocompromised transplant patients, researchers are optimistic that careful inpatient management and close surveillance will lead to infection outcomes that approach those of immunocompetent counterparts.

DISCLOSURE

The authors have nothing to disclose.

REFERENCES

1. Schmidt G, Piponov H, Chuang D, et al. Hand Infections in the Immunocompromised Patient: An Update. J Hand Surg 2019;44(2):144–9.
2. Ching V, Ritz M, Song C, et al. Human immunodeficiency virus infection in an emergency hand service. J Hand Surg 1996;21(4):696–9.
3. Gonzalez MH, Nikoleit J, Weinzweig N, et al. Upper extremity infections in patients with the human immunodeficiency virus. J Hand Surg 1998;23(2):348–52.
4. Houshian S, Seyedipour S, Wedderkopp N. Epidemiology of bacterial hand infections. Int J Infect Dis 2006;10(4):315–9.
5. Camasmie HR, Léda SBCS, Lupi O, et al. Chronic herpetic whitlow as the first manifestation of HIV infection. AIDS 2016;30(14):2254–6.
6. Chan E, Bagg M. Atypical hand infections. OrthopClin North Am 2017;48(2):229–40.
7. Fowler JR. Viral infections. HandClin 1989;5(4):613–27. Available at: https://www.ncbi.nlm.nih.gov/pubmed/2553755.
8. Elhassan BT, Wynn SW, Hand MG. Atypical infections of the hand. 2004. Available at: https://www.sciencedirect.com/science/article/pii/S1531091403001670. Accessed May 10, 2019.
9. Handisurya A, Rieger A, Bankier A, et al. Human papillomavirus type 26 infection causing multiple invasive squamous cell carcinomas of the fingernails in an AIDS patient under highly active antiretroviral therapy. Br J Dermatol 2007;157(4):788–94.
10. Aguayo R, Soria X, Abal L, et al. Bowen's disease associated with human papillomavirus infection of the nail bed. Dermatol Surg 2011;37(1):116–8.
11. Coleman NW, Fleckman P, Huang JI. Fungal nail infections. J Hand Surg 2014;39(5):985–8.
12. Rubright JH, Shafritz AB. The herpetic whitlow. J Hand Surg 2011;36(2):340–2.
13. Gonzalez MH, Bochar S, Novotny J, et al. Upper extremity infections in patients with diabetes mellitus. J Hand Surg 1999;24(4):682–6. Available at: https://www.ncbi.nlm.nih.gov/pubmed/10447157. Accessed July 1, 1999.
14. Sharma K, Pan D, Friedman J, et al. Quantifying the Effect of Diabetes on Surgical Hand and Forearm Infections. J Hand Surg 2018;43(2):105–14.
15. Hostetter MK. Handicaps to host defense. Effects of hyperglycemia on C3 and Candida albicans. Diabetes 1990;39(3):271–5. Available at: https://www.ncbi.nlm.nih.gov/pubmed/2407580.
16. Ferguson BJ. Mucormycosis of the nose and paranasal sinuses. OtolaryngolClin North Am 2000;33(2):349–65. Available at: https://www.ncbi.nlm.nih.gov/pubmed/10736409.
17. Hodgson KA, Morris JL, Feterl ML, et al. Altered macrophage function is associated with severe Burkholderiapseudomallei infection in a murine model of type 2 diabetes. Microbes Infect 2011;13(14–15):1177–84.
18. Stepan JG, Boddapati V, Sacks HA, et al. Insulin Dependence Is Associated With Increased Risk of Complications After Upper Extremity Surgery in Diabetic Patients. J Hand Surg 2018;43(8):745–54.e4.
19. Wong C-H, Chang H-C, Pasupathy S, et al. Necrotizing fasciitis: clinical presentation, microbiology, and determinants of mortality. J Bone Joint Surg Am 2003;85-A(8):1454–60. Available at: https://www.ncbi.nlm.nih.gov/pubmed/12925624.
20. Gonzalez MH. Necrotizing fasciitis and gangrene of the upper extremity. HandClin 1998;14(4):635–45. ix. Available at: https://www.ncbi.nlm.nih.gov/pubmed/9884900.
21. Gaston RG, Kuremsky MA. Postoperative infections: prevention and management. HandClin 2010;26(2):265–80.
22. Osterman M, Draeger R, Stern P. Acute hand infections. J Hand Surg 2014;39(8):1628–35 [quiz: 1635].
23. Fontes RA, Ogilvie CM, Miclau T. Necrotizing soft-tissue infections. J Am AcadOrthop Surg 2000;8(3):151–8. Available at: https://www.ncbi.nlm.nih.gov/pubmed/10874222.
24. Bégon E, Bachmeyer C, Thibault M, et al. Necrotizing fasciitis due to Cryptococcus neoformans in a diabetic patient with chronic renal insufficiency. ClinExpDermatol 2009;34(8):935–6.
25. NeblettFanfair R, Benedict K, Bos J, et al. Necrotizing cutaneous mucormycosis after a tornado in Joplin, Missouri, in 2011. N Engl J Med 2012;367(23):2214–25.
26. Lass-Flörl C. Zygomycosis: conventional laboratory diagnosis. ClinMicrobiol Infect 2009;15(Suppl 5):60–5.
27. Patel MR. Chronic infections. In: Wolfe SW, Hotchkiss RN, Pederson WC, et al, editors. Green's oeprativehand surgery. 7th edition. Philadelphia: Elsevier; 2017. p. 62–127.
28. Moran SL, Strickland J, Shin AY. Upper-extremity mucormycosis infections in immunocompetent patients. J Hand Surg 2006;31(7):1201–5.
29. Jain A, Witbreuk M, Ball C, et al. Influence of steroids and methotrexate on wound complications after elective rheumatoid hand and wrist surgery. J Hand Surg 2002;27(3):449–55. Available at: https://www.ncbi.nlm.nih.gov/pubmed/12015719. Accessed May 1, 2002.

30. Singh JA, Cameron C, Noorbaloochi S, et al. Risk of serious infection in biological treatment of patients with rheumatoid arthritis: a systematic review and meta-analysis. Lancet 2015;386(9990):258–65.

31. Berthold E, Geborek P, Gülfe A. Continuation of TNF blockade in patients with inflammatory rheumatic disease. An observational study on surgical site infections in 1,596 elective orthopedic and hand surgery procedures. ActaOrthop 2013;84(5): 495–501.

32. Al-Qattan MM, Helmi AA. Chronic hand infections. J Hand Surg 2014;39(8):1636–45.

33. Klein MB, Chang J. Management of hand and upper-extremity infections in heart transplant recipients. PlastReconstr Surg 2000;106(3):598–601. Available at: https://www.ncbi.nlm.nih.gov/pubmed/10987466. Accessed September 1, 2000.

34. Francel TJ, Marshall KA, Savage RC. Hand infections in the diabetic and the diabetic renal transplant recipient. Ann Plast Surg 1990;24(4): 304–9. Available at: https://www.ncbi.nlm.nih.gov/pubmed/2353778. Accessed April 1, 1990.

35. Mull AB, Sharma K, Yu JL, et al. Surgical Upper Extremity Infections in Immunosuppressed Patients: A Comparative Analysis With Diagnosis and Treatment Recommendations for Hand Surgeons. Hand 2018. https://doi.org/10.1177/1558944718789410.

36. Goodman SM, Springer B, Guyatt G, et al. 2017 American College of Rheumatology/American Association of Hip and Knee Surgeons Guideline for the Perioperative Management of Antirheumatic Medication in Patients With Rheumatic Diseases Undergoing Elective Total Hip or Total Knee Arthroplasty. ArthritisRheumatol 2017;69(8): 1538–51.

Fungal Infections of the Hand

Mary Patricia Fox, MD*, Sidney M. Jacoby, MD

KEYWORDS

• Fungal infections • Hand • Paronychia • Sporotrichosis

KEY POINTS

- Clinically significant fungal infections of the upper extremity are uncommon. However, the incidence is increasing secondary to an increase in immunocompromised individuals and intentional immunosuppression.
- The most common fungal infections of the hand are cutaneous infections involving the skin and nails.
- Deep fungal infections are rare in the hand and upper extremity but result in serious clinical problems.

OVERVIEW

Clinically significant fungal infections of the upper extremity are uncommon. However, the incidence is increasing secondary to an increase in immuno-compromised individuals, intentional immunosuppression (organ and stem cell transplant), and medicine-induced immunosuppression (chemotherapy, corticosteroid therapy, antibacterial therapy).[1] Fungal infections of the upper extremity are classified based on anatomic location and epidemiology. The anatomic categories that affect the hand include cutaneous, subcutaneous, and deep.[2] Cutaneous infections are caused by organisms that metabolize keratin and can cause serious morbidity but are rarely fatal. Subcutaneous infections are similar to the cutaneous infections and are produced by low-virulence organisms. Cutaneous and subcutaneous infections are most common and can be treated by primary care physicians and dermatologists. Deep infections are far less common but can be fatal without more intensive treatment and are therefore more likely to present to hand surgeons or have the assistance of an upper extremity surgeon as part of a multidisciplinary treatment team.[1,2]

Epidemiologic classifications include endemic and opportunistic infections. The endemic mycoses are caused by fungal organisms acquired from the environment. Soil is the primary source for the endemic mycosis, which are most often acquired by inhalation. These organisms can cause severe infections in immunocompetent patients and fatal infections in immunocompromised patients. Opportunistic fungal infection is typically harmless unless the host immunity is compromised, in which case it may transition to a more invasive pathogen with dire consequences.[1] This article discusses fungal infections related to their typical tissue level of invasion.

CUTANEOUS

The most common fungal infections of the hand are cutaneous infections involving the skin and nails. These infections are caused by fungi that infect and metabolize keratin, termed keratinophilic fungi, and do not invade the body surface. Keratinophilic fungi include fungi from the genera of *Trichophyton*, *Microsporum*, and *Epidermophyton*.[3] The clinical manifestations are a consequence of the host reaction to metabolic

Department of Orthopaedic Surgery, Philadelphia Hand to Shoulder Center, Thomas Jefferson University, 834 Chestnut Street, Suite G-114, Philadelphia, PA 19107, USA
* Corresponding author.
E-mail address: mpgeorge09@gmail.com

Hand Clin 36 (2020) 355–360
https://doi.org/10.1016/j.hcl.2020.03.009

byproducts of the fungal growth.[2] Infections are transmitted by direct contact either by contact with infected individuals or spread from another region of the body.

Trichophyton, the genus of fungi that causes tinea, causes the most common cutaneous infection. Its characteristic clinical presentation includes red, scaly, concentric rings in the affected area, commonly referred to as ringworm. The skin disease can be seen on the dorsum of the hand and in interdigital spaces. Tinea nigra is a special form of tinea that is caused by pigmented organisms other than *Trichophyton*. The typical organism is *Exophiala werneckii* and is common in hot humid environments such as the topics and in the southern or coastal regions of the United States. Tinea nigra presents with a darkened patch of skin that can be confused for melanoma or nevus.[1,2]

Candida albicans can also cause cutaneous infections and is most commonly seen in moist skin. It may be seen in patients with spasticity presenting with clenched fists.[1]

Fungal infection of the nails, onychomycosis, is more common in the feet than in the hands and is caused by *Trichophyton rubrum*. Discoloration of the nail with asymmetrical changes are the primary clinical manifestations of onychomycosis (**Fig. 1**). The nail changes of psoriasis can be confused with onychomycosis but are often symmetric nail changes as opposed to asymmetric respectively.[2,4]

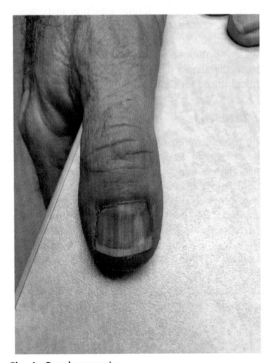

Fig. 1. Onychomycosis.

Diagnosis

Most of the cutaneous fungi are easily identified by the demonstration of septated hyphae and spores from the skin or nail scrapings of the suspected area on a wet KOH preparation under microscope review. Occasionally definitive diagnoses are required with fungal cultures on Sabouraud medium to distinguish between *Trichophyton* and *C albicans*.[1,3]

Treatment

Uncomplicated cases of trichophytosis can be treated with topical cream or lotions such as tolnaftate (Tinactin), miconazole (Monistat), or ciclopirox (Loprox) for 2 to 3 weeks. More widespread lesions may require oral antifungals such as ketoconazole, fluconazole, itraconazole, or griseofulvin.[1–3] Of clinical note, the use of oral antifungals requires close monitoring of liver function tests on a monthly basis, because of hepatic clearance. This monitoring requires close involvement of the primary care team to monitor both pharmacologic cross reactivity and overall liver function.

C albicans can be treated by keeping the affected area clean and dry combined with topical nystatin ointment. In patients with spasticity, surgical management may be warranted, including tendon lengthening, which may prevent recurrent infections if local hand hygiene fails.

Onychomycosis rarely resolves spontaneously. Topical treatment with ciclopirox or gentian violet is an option for patients that have contraindications to the oral antifungals. Oral antifungals such as ketoconazole or terbinafine must be taken for long durations and can cause significant side effects. Surgical removal of the nail followed by topical therapy can also be effective. In addition, marsupialization of the skin proximal to the eponychial nail fold or surgical removal of the nail with nail bed ablation is an option with high cure rates.[2,4]

SUBCUTANEOUS

The 2 major subcutaneous fungal infections of the hand are chronic paronychia and sporotrichosis.[1,2]

Chronic Paronychia

Chronic paronychia is seen as a well-localized area of skin inflammation at the proximal nail fold. The cuticle is retracted, rounded, and detached from the nail plate. This alteration in cuticle anatomy allows a pocket of water to become entrapped under the proximal nail fold. The retention of water allows fungus to thrive in this environment. It may initially be misdiagnosed as a bacterial infection with lack of response to usual antibiotics. It affects patients who frequently soak their hands in water and can be seen from mechanical trauma from nail salons. *C albicans* is primary cause of chronic paronychia (70%–97% of cases).[1–3]

The initial changes begin at the lateral nail fold with chronic swelling and separation of the fold from the margin. It progresses to the eponychium and the cuticle separates from the nail plate, allowing the moisture to reside and creating an environment for *C albicans*. As the process progresses, the germinal matrix is invaded, which results in irregularities in the nail plate, such as grooving. The nail plate can become greenish because of secondary colonization of *Pseudomonas aeruginosa*.[1]

Diagnosis is primarily based on clinical manifestation with the characteristic nail fold changes of chronically indurated, retracted, rounded eponychium. Most affected individuals are women with a long history of disfigured thickening of the eponychial skin. If necessary, skin and nail scrapings can be used to identify *C albicans* by culture.

Treatment includes keeping the area as dry as possible with application of an antifungal agent such as clotrimazole. A more effective option is treatment with an oral antifungal such as fluconazole. However, both topical and oral treatment remain frustrating with limited success, as shown by 40% of treated individuals remaining free of infection.[1] When conservative management fails, surgical management, including marsupialization of the affected area, should be considered. This technique involves excising a symmetric, crescent-shaped segment of skin, leaving a bridge of skin proximal to the eponychium. The nail should be removed when nail irregularities are present.[5]

Sporotrichosis

Sporotrichosis is caused by the dimorphic fungus *Sporothrix schenckii* and is the most common lymphocutaneous fungal infection in North America. Most cases are reported from the Missouri and Mississippi Rivers and the fungus is found in the soil. The *Sporothrix* spore is inoculated into the skin and deeper tissues by a rose thorn, hence rose-thorn or rose-gardeners' disease. The infection is seen as an occupational hazard of those working on gardens or farms.[1,2,6]

The inoculation produces a chronic granulomatous infection with a primary ulcerative lesion at the site of infection and secondary ascending lymphadenopathy. The infected lymph node develops a characteristic violet ulceration and drains seropurulent fluid, which can be cultured. Cultures are grown on modified Sabouraud agar, incubated at 30°C or room temperature, and are positive after a few days. Examination of biopsy specimens reveals a pyogranulomatous response with the characteristic cigar-shaped yeast.

The treatment of choice for sporotrichosis is itraconazole, 200 mg/d for 3 to 6 months. The traditional treatment of choice was a saturated solution of potassium iodide, 1 g/mL at a dose of 3 to 4 g orally 3 times a day for 6 to 8 weeks. Side effects include gastrointestinal distress, skin rashes, and thyroid dysfunction. This treatment is inexpensive and effective and is still a mainstay of treatment in developing countries.[3]

DEEP

Deep fungal infections are rare in the hand and upper extremity but result in serious clinical problems. These infections can present with both superficial and deep components, and fungal stains and cultures are necessary to make a diagnosis. In addition, a multidisciplinary approach is warranted, with consultation of infectious disease specialists for management of drug therapy.

Aspergillosis

Aspergillus infections are seen in immunocompromised patients and occur as localized dermal necrotic nodules. They are most commonly caused by *Aspergillus fumigatus* and are a major cause of morbidity, including hand amputation, and mortality secondary to infecting blood vessels and causing tissue necrosis. Risk factors to be aware of are infections associated with burns and intravenous or catheter sites.[7,8]

Diagnosis is obtained from biopsy of necrotic lesions showing numerous fungal hyphae on a wet KOH preparation.

Treatment is difficult and comprehensive, with radical surgical debridement, antifungal drug therapy, and reduction of immunosuppressive therapy. Serial debridements may be necessary secondary to invasiveness and devastating tissue necrosis. Intravenous or oral voriconazole is the drug of choice and has replaced amphotericin B because it is more potent and has fewer side effects. Excision of the lesion is the treatment of choice in immunocompetent patients.

Blastomycosis

Blastomycosis is endemic in North America's Ohio River and Mississippi River valleys and is caused by *Blastomyces dermatitidis*. It occurs in both immunocompromised and immunocompetent hosts. It primarily affects hosts who work in contact with the soil, which can cause direct implantation of the fungus into the skin and lead to primary cutaneous blastomycosis. Cutaneous blastomycosis is the most common presenting sign of the disease. This condition can be seen in veterinarians who have handled an infected animal. Blastomycosis can also be inhaled and cause lung infection, and, in turn, the fungus can spread from the lungs into the skin and cause cutaneous blastomycosis.[1,3]

Unlike sporotrichosis, with characteristic ascending lymphadenopathy and ulcers, the clinical manifestations for blastomycosis are nonspecific. A high clinical suspicion is warranted. The skin lesion may appear as a plaque, ulcer, or nodule; may be isolated or multiple; and can be found throughout the hand and upper extremity. The dorsum of the hand is a common location. Nodules can develop into abscesses with draining fistulas and then into ulcers. Furthermore, spread to tendon, joint, and bone can be seen in 60% of patients with the systemic form. Lesions around the joints present in patients with systemic blastomycosis and can lead to septic arthritis and osteomyelitis.[1,3]

Diagnosis is made from a biopsy of the affected tissue and requires special stains, such as periodic acid–Schiff or silver stain. The characteristic histologic appearance seen with blastomycosis is a double refractile cell wall and broad-based buds between the mother and daughter cells.

Treatment of both cutaneous and systemic forms includes systemic antifungal with ketoconazole or itraconazole. Surgical debulking is questionable.

Candidiasis

Fungal infections caused by the *Candida* genus are most commonly seen in both cutaneous and subcutaneous infections but can cause deep infections. *Candida* are opportunist fungi when causing deep infections and are seen in vulnerable populations. Local and systemic candidiasis is seen in the human immunodeficiency virus population, with prosthetic devices, and in newborns. The most common species recovered from clinical specimens include *C albicans*, *Candida tropicalis*, *Candida glabrata*, and *Candida parapsilosis*.

Clinical manifestations can range from interdigital web ulcers, flexor and/or extensor tenosynovitis, septic arthritis, osteomyelitis, and periprosthetic infections such as infection of silicone arthroplasty of the metacarpophalangeal joint.

Diagnosis includes aspiration of affected joint and surgical debridement for biopsy tissue. Staining and culture for the fungus should be included.

Treatment of choice includes systemic antifungals, fluconazole, and amphotericin B. Surgical debridement, radical synovectomy, and removal of implant is necessary for periprosthetic infections. Surgical debridement is also necessary for flexor and/or extensor tenosynovitis, septic arthritis, and osteomyelitis.[1,3]

Coccidioidomycosis

Coccidioidomycosis is a rare fungal infection that is endemic to the hot and arid regions of the San Joaquin Valley in California and the US deserts of the southwest. It is caused by *Coccidioides immitis*.

Coccidioidal infections occur in the wrist and hand and have a predilection for synovium. Patients present with diffuse swelling either on the dorsal or volar side of the wrist or palm. It can lead to extensor tendon rupture and thus mimic rheumatoid arthritis. The most common presentation of deep coccidioidal infection in the hand is osteomyelitis with a predilection for the ends of long bones and bony prominences.[6]

Diagnosis is made from identification of *C immitis* in synovial stains and cultures. The excised tissue shows the classic spherules in synovium and dimorphic fungus in culture. In addition, complement fixation titer is positive.

Treatment of coccidioidomycosis is considered difficult and prolonged secondary to the multiple recurrences and long duration of medical management. An infectious disease consultant is highly recommended because of the long-term commitment to therapy, which includes knowing the side effects and drug interactions. The treatment modalities of choice include surgical radical synovectomy; tenosynovectomy; curettage; and systemic antifungals, such as fluconazole, itraconazole, and amphotericin B.

Cryptococcosis

Cryptococcosis is associated with pigeons and pigeon droppings and can be a devastating disease in the immunocompromised population. There are 2 varieties: *Cryptococcus neoformans* and *Cryptococcus gattii*. *C neoformans* is an opportunistic fungus and, in immunocompromised patients, starts in the lung and disseminates to other sites, including the lungs, central nervous system, and thirdly the skin. In immunocompetent patients, primary lung infection is rare and is typically asymptomatic and resolves.

Cutaneous cryptococcosis manifests in several different ways, which include papules, pustules, plaques, cellulitis, nodules, abscesses, sinuses, and ulcers. All skin manifestations can result in treatment problems for hand surgeons. Case reports have identified *C neoformans* as a cause for tenosynovitis. Vulnerable populations, such patients with as end-stage renal disease, diabetes, malignancy, and medicine-induced immunosuppression, are most at risk to this fungus. In addition, cryptococcosis is an acquired immunodeficiency syndrome–defining disease. Thick and tenacious pus in the wound should arouse suspicion of cryptococcosis. Cryptococcosis has been reported as presenting with osteomyelitis of the digit. Plain films show a lytic lesion with or without a periosteal reaction.[1–3]

Diagnosis is made with tissue biopsy and fluids from sinus, ulcer, or abscess. India ink is mixed with the fluid or tissue and identifies capsulated yeast and granulomatous inflammation. Diagnosis can be confirmed by a high cryptococcal antigen titer and subsequent growth on culture.

The recommended treatment regimen includes systemic antifungal with amphotericin B with flucytosine. An alternative treatment is fluconazole or itraconazole. Surgical management is an adjunctive treatment depending on the clinical presentation.

Histoplasmosis

Histoplasmosis is associated with bat and cat feces and is endemic to the Ohio River and Mississippi River valleys. Histoplasmosis is caused by *Histoplasma capsulatum*. It is contracted by inhalation and is a pulmonary pathogen. In immunocompetent hosts, the disease is subclinical and self-limiting; however, in immunocompromised patients it can lead to disseminated disease.

Clinical manifestation includes cutaneous infection, tendon ruptures, tenosynovitis, arthritis, and necrotizing myofascitis. The infected synovial tissue is red-brown, contains rice bodies, and undergoes active caseous granulomatous inflammation.

Disseminated histoplasmosis may present with fever and weight loss and can have a high mortality when not treated in a timely manner.

Diagnosis is difficult because it is difficult to isolate *H capsulatum* from clinical specimens. Grocott silver stain is needed for the biopsy and shows large, round, single-celled spores, and serology testing is used for complement fixation of antibodies. A titer of 1:8 is considered presumptive and a titer of 1:32 is significantly suggestive of active infection.[1,6]

Treatment of choice includes surgical and medical management with a combination of tenosynovectomy, bone debridement, and systemic antifungal therapy with either ketoconazole or intravenous amphotericin B.

Mucormycosis

Mucormycosis is caused by the fungi of the class Mucoromycotina and order Mucorales. The most common pathogens isolated are *Rhizopus* species, followed by *Rhizomucor*.[9] Despite the name, *Mucor* species are a rare cause of mucormycosis. Mucormycosis is caused by these opportunistic fungi and can result in a devastating disease in both the immunocompetent and immunocompromised hosts. Similar to *Aspergillus*, infection is characterized by vascular infection, arterial and venous thrombosis, and gangrenous tissue infarction and necrosis. This infection rapidly disseminates into the local blood vessels at the site of infection and quickly spreads to adjacent soft tissue and bone. It is aggressive and relentless and has a higher morbidity and mortality than other fungal infections, greater than 40%. This rate approached 80% in the presence of necrotizing fasciitis.[1] Mechanism of spread includes external implantation in the setting of heavy soil contamination in open wounds and penetrating injury from plant material.[10] It has been seen from catheter insertion, injections of medications such as insulin or steroids, and use of tape to secure oxygen-monitoring devices.

Infection of the hand is usually cutaneous or subcutaneous, and an isolated lesion can occur anywhere from the hand to the shoulder. The lesions are black skin eschars and gangrene. It has been described in 3 stages: dermal plexus (black eschar), subcutaneous vessels (bleeding ulcer), and deep extension to major arteries (digital and hand gangrene). In immunocompetent patients, clinical suspicion should be high in patients with severe trauma who sustained a large open wound that is heavily contaminated by soil, as seen in high-energy automobile and agriculture injuries. In immunodeficient patients, most have diabetes, chronic kidney failure, organ transplants, and/or leukemia. An infection may occur from simple trauma, such as intravenous or arterial line sites.[1,9,10]

Diagnosis is first based on clinical suspicion given the speed of the infection. Mucormycosis is a triad of rapid cutaneous and subcutaneous gangrenous destruction, diabetes, and blood vessel thrombosis. The clinical manifestations of enlarging black skin eschars and gangrene should lead to the diagnosis of mucormycosis. If it is suspected, there is an urgent need for biopsy. Biopsy and histology remain the most sensitive and specific options for definitive diagnosis. Tissue biopsy confirms the diagnosis with 90° hyphae visualized in a 10% KOH stain.

Treatment includes rapid diagnosis and radical debridement of all necrotic tissues. A systemic antifungal should be started immediately and the drug of choice is a high-dose lipid formulation of amphotericin B. In addition, any predisposing risks factors or immunosuppressive medications should be reduced or stopped.

SUMMARY

Fungal infections of the hand are most commonly cutaneous infections involving the skin and nails and can be treated with topical or local therapy. However, deep fungal infections can cause severe morbidity and even mortality, and clinicians should maintain a high level of suspicion in patients with presenting lesions and predisposing risks factors. A timely diagnosis is the most important factor for successful management.

DISCLOSURE

The authors have nothing to disclose.

REFERENCES

1. Patel MR. Chronic infections. In: Wolfe SW, Hotchkiss RN, Pederson W, et al, editors. Green's operative hand surgery, vol 1, 7th edition. Philadelphia: Elsevier; 2017. p. 62–127.
2. Amadio PC. Fungal infection of the hand. Hand Clin 1998;14(4):605–12.
3. Chan E, Bagg M. Atypical hand infections. Orthop Clin North Am 2017;48:229–40.
4. Franko OI, Abrams RA. Hand infections. Orthop Clin North Am 2013;44:625–34.
5. Keyser JJ, Littler JW, Eaton RG. Surgical treatment of infections and lesions of the perionychium. Hand Clin 1990;6(1):137–53.
6. Mohammad AM, Helmi AA. Chronic hand infections. J Hand Surg Am 2014;39(8):1636–45.
7. Jones NF, Conklin WT, Albdo VC. Primary invasive aspergillosis of the hand. J Hand Surg Am 1986; 11(3):425–8.
8. Olorunnipa O, Zhang AY, Curtin CM. Invasive aspergillosis of the hand caused by Aspergillus ustus: a case report. Hand (N Y) 2010;5(1):102–5.
9. Fathi P, Vranis NM, Paryavi E. Diagnosis and treatment of upper extremity Mucormycosis infection. J Hand Surg Am 2015;40(5):1032–4.
10. Moran SL, Strickland J, Shin AY. Upper-extremity Mucormycosis infections in immunocompetent patients. J Hand Surg Am 2006;31A:1201–5.

Complications of Hand Infections

Joshua Luginbuhl, MD, Mark K. Solarz, MD*

KEYWORDS

- Hand infections • Complications • Stiffness • Diabetes • Osteomyelitis • Immunocompromised

KEY POINTS

- Hand infections are associated with a high rate of complications that are often difficult to manage.
- Risk factors for the development of complications from hand infections include a history of diabetes mellitus, an immunocompromised state, and a delay in presentation.
- Common complications include osteomyelitis, which frequently results in amputation, stiffness requiring therapy or tenolysis, and soft tissue defects requiring complex wound management.

INTRODUCTION

There are a wide variety of commonly encountered infections that affect the hand. Infections can be isolated to the finger, as is seen in paronychia, felon, herpetic whitlow, and pyogenic flexor tenosynovitis, or can involve the deep spaces of the hand. In most cases, appropriate treatment results in eradication of the infection and return to baseline function. However, complications of hand infections are encountered frequently. These complications can include osteomyelitis, stiffness, and soft tissue defects, and in most cases they are more difficult to treat than the initial infection. Risk factors that predispose patients to the development of complications during the treatment of hand infections include diabetes mellitus, an immunocompromised state resulting from an underlying medical condition or medication, and delay in presentation.

RISK FACTORS
Diabetes

Diabetes mellitus is a prevalent medical condition that ultimately leads to an immunocompromised state. High glucose levels cause decreased neutrophil synthesis. Additionally, cytosolic calcium increases in the presence of hyperglycemia and is inversely proportional to phagocytic activity.[1] Besides the detrimental effects it has on the body's innate immunity, high blood glucose also damages nerves and microvascular structures, which lead to peripheral neuropathy and decrease oxygen delivery to tissues, respectively.[2] When combined, the negative effects of diabetes on peripheral nerves, blood vessels, and neutrophils can lead to delayed wound healing and reduced ability to prevent infection (**Fig. 1**).

Patients with diabetes are at a higher risk of developing more severe hand infections, likely related to the often polymicrobial nature of their infections and diminished host immune response.[3–6] A study by Jalil and colleagues[4] found that 41% of hand infections in patients with diabetes are caused by more than 1 organism, making appropriate antibiotic selection more challenging. Hand infections caused by fungus and yeast are also more common in patients with diabetes with an incidence of 10.3% and 9.0%, respectively.[4] Because these organisms often require a longer period of time to be positively identified by culture when compared with aerobic and anaerobic bacteria, correct antibiotic administration is frequently delayed.

Department of Orthopaedics and Sports Medicine, Temple University Hospital, 3401 North Broad Street, Philadelphia, PA 19140, USA
* Corresponding author.
E-mail address: mark.solarz@tuhs.temple.edu

Hand Clin 36 (2020) 361–367
https://doi.org/10.1016/j.hcl.2020.03.010
0749-0712/20/© 2020 Elsevier Inc. All rights reserved.

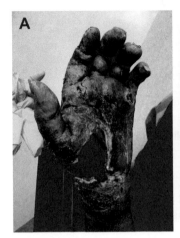 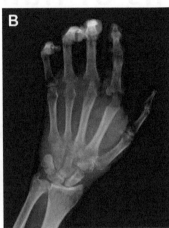

Fig. 1. (*A*, *B*) Complicated hand infection in a patient with diabetes, including pyogenic flexor tenosynovitis and volar skin necrosis along with underlying osteomyelitis.

Several studies have demonstrated an overall higher complication rate and poorer outcomes in the treatment of hand infections in those with a history of diabetes mellitus, estimated to be as high as 60.0% compared with 10.7% in patients without diabetes.[4,5,7–10] Deep space infections and polymicrobial infections, each known to be more commonly seen in patients with diabetes, are associated with increased length of hospital stay, reoperation, and amputation.[4]

When comparing hand infections in patients with and without diabetes, infections associated with diabetes are more likely to result from an idiopathic mechanism, occur in the forearm, and present as osteomyelitis, septic arthritis, or necrotizing fasciitis as reported by Sharma and collegues.[8] The need for repeat drainage is associated with poor glycemic control, defined as glycosylated hemoglobin of 9.0% or greater and poor inpatient control of blood glucose (>180 mg/dL).[8]

In a series of 45 consecutive patients with diabetes with 46 upper extremity infections, Gonzalez and colleagues[3] found that 50% of patients required more than one operation, 39% required amputation, and 3 patients died from causes considered to be directly related to their infection. When an anaerobic organism was isolated, 6 of the 7 cases required amputation. In another series of 50 patients with diabetes with hand infections, the amputation rate was 17.5% when an abscess was present.[7] **Fig. 1** shows a patient with an extensive upper extremity that ultimately required amputation.

A significant portion of upper extremity infections occur in patients with diabetes. Complications in patients with diabetes, although more common than in the general population, can be prevented with a multidisciplinary approach using proper glycemic control, elevation of the extremity, thorough and adequate surgical debridement, and appropriate antibiotic therapy.[4]

Immunocompromised patients

Patients in relatively immunocompromised states are becoming more commonly encountered by the hand surgeon. The rate of human immunodeficiency virus (HIV) infection is expected to increase with the current opioid epidemic. In 2015, the number of HIV diagnoses attributed to intravenous drug use increased for the first time in 2 decades.[11] In recent years, there has also been an increase in the number of immunocompromised patients owing to the development of immunosuppressive medications for both transplant recipients and those with autoimmune disorders. Despite the benefits of these medications in improving quality of life, they do place these patients at higher risk for the development of infections and subsequent complications from these infections.

Human immunodeficiency virus

According to a 2017 report by the Centers for Disease Control and Prevention, the prevalence of HIV has increased in the United States. Patients with the virus have longer life expectancies owing to advancements in antiretroviral therapies, and transmission is increasing along with the increase in intravenous drug use during the current opioid epidemic.[11] HIV compromises the immune system by interfering with T cells and the adaptive immunity. As a result, patients with the virus are at increased risk of hand infections from nonpenetrating trauma. Similar to patients who have a competent immune system, the most common pathogen is *Staphylococcus aureus*.[12]

In a study of hand infections in 24 patients with HIV, Ching and colleagues[12] revealed that HIV reactivity was associated with longer hospital stays and more surgical procedures. These findings may be related to the higher incidence, up to 6-fold, of methicillin-resistant *S aureus* causing soft tissue infections in HIV-infected patients when compared with patients without HIV.[13]

Additionally, those with HIV may have an atypical and/or more severe presentation of common hand infections. Herpetic whitlow, which is caused by herpes simplex virus 1 and 2, may completely destroy the nail bed in patients who are significantly immunocompromised. These vulnerable patients need to be treated quickly and definitively and may require oral or intravenous antiviral therapy.[2]

Immunosuppressive medications

Immunosuppressive medications have revolutionized the treatment of autoimmune disorders such as rheumatoid arthritis and are used after solid organ transplantation to avoid rejection, improving the lives of countless individuals. Despite their benefits, these medications do place patients at risk for developing severe infections and subsequent complications.

In a series reviewing 911 cardiac transplant recipients, Klein and Chang[14] found that 13 patients were treated for hand infections and 10 of those infections required operative debridement. Three of the 10 required multiple trips to the operating room and, when compared with nonimmunosuppressed patients, cardiac transplant recipients were more likely to present with deep space infection, tenosynovitis, and osteomyelitis.[14] More than one-half of these patients had a polymicrobial infection, 4 of the 13 patients (31%) had a fungal infection, and 1 had a mycobacterial infection.[14]

Complications occur at a very high rate and are associated with poor outcomes when hand infections occur in renal transplant recipients with a history of diabetes. The amputation rate for patients in a series by Francel and colleagues[10] was 100% with an average of 3.8 digits per patient. These patients were hospitalized for an average of 41.2 days.[10] This finding is a stark comparison when comparing nontransplant patients, whose amputation rate was 51.6% with an average amputation of 1.2 digits per patient. Not surprisingly, length of stay was also shorter in these patients at 15.2 days.[10]

Similar to medical management after solid organ transplantation, the treatment of autoimmune disorders often involves medications that deliberately weaken the immune system. In the last few decades, disease-modifying antirheumatic drugs have gained popularity in controlling the disease process of rheumatoid arthritis in addition to other autoimmune conditions.

In a study of 129 surgical procedures of the hand and wrist involving patients with rheumatoid arthritis, there was no significantly increased risk of wound infection in patients taking steroids or methotrexate through the perioperative period.[15] Likewise, Berthold and colleagues[16] reviewed the difference in soft tissue infection when tumor necrosis factor inhibitors were continued or discontinued around the time of elective orthopedic surgery in 1551 patients and found a significant increase of complications only in the foot and ankle group. There was no increase in infection rate in the hand surgery cohort.[16]

Despite these encouraging results with regard to elective hand procedures, anti-tumor necrosis factor medications were associated with an increased risk of delayed wound healing and early postoperative wound infections after orthopedic procedures in another study.[17] The American College of Rheumatology and the American Association of Hip and Knee Surgeons recommend pausing treatment with anti-tumor necrosis factor agents in the perioperative period. They recommend scheduling surgery at the end of the dosing cycle for these specific medications and restarting the medication once wound healing has occurred.[18]

Like patients who are immunosuppressed owing to diabetes or HIV, hand infections in those whose immune systems are medically compromised require early identification and aggressive treatment to limit complications.

Delay in Presentation

Delayed presentation of hand infections often leads to a more complicated clinical picture, which in turn leads to more difficulty eradicating the infection. Frequently the delay in presentation is patient related, however, occasionally it is owing to infection with a less typical causative organism, most notably fungal infections.[19]

A delay in presentation often leads to extensive destruction of the native anatomy (**Fig. 2**). For example, a delay in treatment of septic arthritis of the proximal interphalangeal joint can lead to osteomyelitis and a boutonniere deformity owing to disruption of the extensor mechanism.[20] Additionally, those presenting late may have more soft tissue and skin damage, which would in turn increase the likelihood of multiple surgical procedures including soft tissue coverage of the defect.

In a retrospective study of 379 patients with hand infections, a delay in surgical intervention of more than 1 day extended the hospital stay by 1.22 days.[21] Overall, late presentation leads to longer inpatient hospital stays and a higher number of surgical procedures, which are often

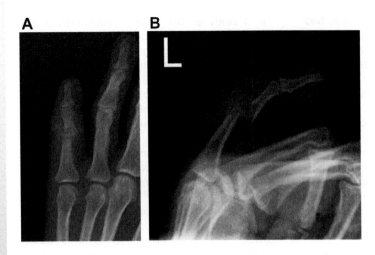

Fig. 2. (A, B). Delayed presentation of proximal interphalangeal joint septic arthritis with osseous destruction owing to osteomyelitis.

necessary to account for the complications such as osteomyelitis, tendon rupture, stiffness, and soft tissue defects (**Fig. 3**).

COMPLICATIONS
Osteomyelitis

Osteomyelitis is a pyogenic infection of the bone. It can occur from direct inoculation, spread from adjacent tissues, or hematogenously. When a sequestrum develops, it is nearly impossible to eradicate the infection with antibiotic therapy alone owing to the hypovascularity and poor antibiotic penetration.[22]

In a review of 700 patients with hand infections, Reilly and colleagues[23] reported that 7% of patients eventually developed osteomyelitis of the metacarpals or phalangeal bones. Most commonly, in 57% of cases the infection was caused by direct trauma. Hematogenous spread was the cause in 13% of cases and spread from

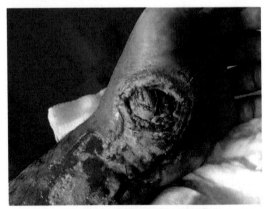

Fig. 3. Delayed presentation of a complicated volar hand abscess in a patient with a history of intravenous drug use.

contiguous infections occurred in 9% of patients.[23]

The workup for osteomyelitis typically consists of serologic inflammatory markers, plain radiographs (see **Fig. 3**), and MRI. Bone biopsy and culture remain the gold standard for diagnosis.[24,25]

Eradication of osteomyelitis in the hand requires surgical debridement of the involved bone and culture-guided antibiotic therapy often for 4 to 6 weeks.[26,27] Cultures taken during bone debridement in osteomyelitis positively identified an organism in 74% of patients in 1 study. Thirty-five percent of positive cultures were polymicrobial, 35% were gram positive, 15% were gram negative, 12% were fungal infection, and 3% were caused by mycobacterium.[23] Antimicrobials should be bactericidal, parenteral, and cover for both gram-positive and gram-negative organisms empirically until culture-guided therapy is possible.[22]

Once the diagnosis of osteomyelitis in the hand has been confirmed, treatment involves excision of the involved bone. The rate of amputation is particularly high if there is a delay in treatment. In 1 study, those presenting more than 6 months from onset of symptoms had an amputation rate of 86%.[23]

Although amputations are commonly performed when treating osteomyelitis of the hand, more sophisticated surgeries for the treatment of osteomyelitis have also been described. Hara and colleagues[28] reported the use of the Masquelet technique to reconstruct a proximal interphalangeal joint that had been destroyed by osteomyelitis. Additionally, Aimé and colleagues[29] describe 12 patients (13 digits) who had joint-spanning, antibiotic eluting methyl methacrylate spacers placed as definitive single stage treatment for digital osteomyelitis. They reported that 10 of 13 infections were successfully treated at 24 months.

One patient required a second operation to revise a soft tissue flap, but the spacer remained in place.[29]

Osteomyelitis is a common complication in hand infections and is typically treated with surgical debridement and culture-guided antibiotic administration. Although amputation of the involved digits is commonly performed, more innovative management techniques do exist.

Stiffness

With soft tissue infections of the hand, normal digital motion is often limited by pain and edema. Local tissues are damaged by the infectious process and healing can result in arthrofibrosis or tendon adhesions. Therefore, patients with hand infections are at risk for developing significant stiffness despite expedient surgical treatment and proper antibiotic therapy.[30]

In a review of 69 patients with pyogenic flexor tenosynovitis, patients regained two-thirds of their baseline digital motion on average at 6 weeks after surgical treatment and 81% of full motion at 30 months postoperatively.[31] Basadre and colleagues[32] found that, although patients with hand infections owing to human bites lost motion and grip strength if surgical debridement was not performed, patients who presented within 1 to 7 days and underwent incision and drainage had overall good outcomes.

Pang and colleagues[5] reported on recovery of motion following hand infections stratified into 3 groups by severity of infection. Group I had no subcutaneous purulence or digital ischemia. In this group, there were no amputations and recovered a mean 80% return of total active motion. Group II was defined as the presence of subcutaneous purulence but no ischemic changes, and there was an average 72% recovery of motion. The most severe group had both purulence and ischemic changes present. Not surprisingly, these patients had the worst outcomes with recovery of only 49% active range of motion.[5] From these results, it can be concluded that the more severe the hand infection, the more likely the patient is to develop significant motion deficits.

It is critical that patients with hand infections who undergo surgical treatment receive hand therapy postoperatively to maximize range of motion. In patients with persistent hand stiffness despite an appropriate course of hand therapy, extensor and/or flexor tenolysis can be performed to restore active range of motion. Ideally, surgery is performed after the tissues are absent of inflammation and passive motion exceeds active motion.[5]

Soft Tissue Defect

Severe hand infections may result in skin and soft tissue defects that are not amenable to closure. Typically, these large defects are the result of delayed presentation and necessary surgical debridement (**Fig. 4**). In some instances, these wounds can be managed by tertiary or delayed primary closure when amenable. However, in other instances these defects may require skin grafting or soft tissue transfer. The first step in successfully covering a soft tissue defect is eradication of the infection. This procedure may require serial debridements, negative pressure wound therapy, or a combination of both.

An acellular bilaminate membrane by Integra Life Sciences (Princeton, NJ) has gained popularity as a coverage option for an incompetent dermis, which can be seen after severe hand infections. It consists of a porous surface of cross-lined bovine tendon collage and chrondroitin-6-6 sulfate and has been shown to facilitate migration of fibroblasts, macrophages, lymphocytes, and capillary ingrowth to effectively regenerate the dermis.[33] Although the neodermis created can epithelialize over time, it is often used in combination with split thickness skin grafts to expedite coverage (**Fig. 5**).

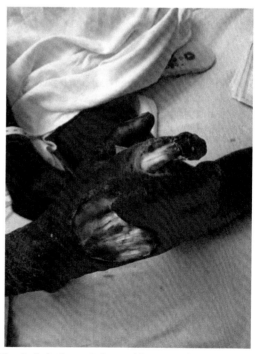

Fig. 4. Soft tissue defects with exposed extensor tendons of the dorsal hand and index finger in a patient with uncontrolled diabetes mellitus after multiple surgical debridements.

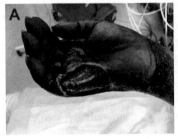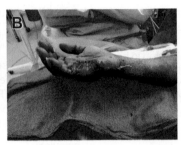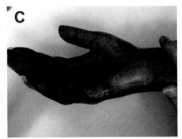

Fig. 5. (*A*) Soft tissue defect after multiple debridements of a volar hand abscess in a patient with uncontrolled diabetes mellitus. (*B*) The wound was covered with Integra dermal template and (*C*) allowed to epithelialize.

Reynolds and colleagues[34] reported the use of an Integra dermal template in the management of complex hand wounds from cancer resection and nonburn trauma in 14 patients. In their study, the mean defect size was 19 cm². Seventy-nine percent of patients had exposed tendon without peritenon, 43% had exposed bone without periosteum, and 28% had exposed joint capsule. The mean time from Integra placement to skin graft was 11.3 days, and negative-pressure wound therapy did not significantly decrease the mean time from placement. Good results were achieved; 13 patients achieved successful reconstruction and, at 6 months postoperatively, 92% patients had return of preoperative hand function. They also found that 85% of patients were extremely satisfied with the aesthetic result and 15% were fairly satisfied.[34]

SUMMARY

Hand infections are common but can be difficult to treat, particularly in those who have diabetes, are immunocompromised, or delay presentation. There is a high incidence of complications such as osteomyelitis, stiffness, and soft tissue defects seen in this population. Patients who develop complications from a hand infection should be treated quickly and aggressively with a multidisciplinary team to prevent further complications and reduce patient morbidity and mortality.

DISCLOSURE

The authors have nothing to disclose.

REFERENCES

1. Alexiewicz JM, Kumar D, Smogorzewski M, et al. Polymorphonuclear leukocytes in non-insulin-dependent diabetes mellitus: abnormalities in metabolism and function. Ann Intern Med 1995;123(12):919–24.

2. Schmidt G, Piponov H, Chuang D, et al. Hand infections in the immunocompromised patient: an update. J Hand Surg Am 2019;44(2):144–9.

3. Gonzalez MH, Bochar S, Novotny J, et al. Upper extremity infections in patients with diabetes mellitus. J Hand Surg Am 1999;24(4):682–6.

4. Jalil A, Barlaan PI, Fung BKK, et al. Hand infection in diabetic patients. Hand Surg 2011;16(03):307–12.

5. Pang H-N, Teoh L-C, Yam AKT, et al. Factors affecting the prognosis of pyogenic flexor tenosynovitis. J Bone Joint Surg 2007;89(8):1742–8.

6. Mandel MA. Immune competence and diabetes mellitus: pyogenic human hand infections. J Hand Surg Am 1978;3(5):458–61.

7. Connor RW, Kimbrough RC, Dabezies EJ. Hand infections in patients with diabetes mellitus. Orthopedics 2001;24(11):1057–60.

8. Sharma K, Pan D, Friedman J, et al. Quantifying the effect of diabetes on surgical hand and forearm infections. J Hand Surg Am 2018;43(2):105–14.

9. Houshian S, Seyedipour S, Wedderkopp N. Epidemiology of bacterial hand infections. Int J Infect Dis 2006;10(4):315–9.

10. Francel TJ, Marshall KA, Savage RC. Hand infections in the diabetic and the diabetic renal transplant recipient. Ann Plast Surg 1990;24(4):304–9.

11. Centers for Disease Control and Prevention. NCHHSTP AtlasPlus. 2017. Available at: https://www.cdc.gov/nchhstp/atlas/index.htm. Accessed June 1, 2019.

12. Ching V, Ritz M, Song C, et al. Human immunodeficiency virus infection in an emergency hand service. J Hand Surg Am 1996;21(4):696–9.

13. Popovich KJ, Weinstein RA, Aroutcheva A, et al. Community-associated methicillin-resistant Staphylococcus aureus and HIV: intersecting epidemics. Clin Infect Dis 2010;50(7):979–87.

14. Klein MB, Chang J. Management of hand and upper-extremity infections in heart transplant recipients. Plast Reconstr Surg 2000;106(3):598–601.

15. Jain A, Witbreuk M, Ball C, et al. Influence of steroids and methotrexate on wound complications after elective rheumatoid hand and wrist surgery. J Hand Surg Am 2002;27(3):449–55.

16. Berthold E, Geborek P, Gülfe A. Continuation of TNF blockade in patients with inflammatory rheumatic disease. An observational study on surgical site infections in 1,596 elective orthopedic and hand surgery procedures. Acta Orthop 2013;84(5):495–501.

17. Giles JT, Bartlett SJ, Gelber AC. Tumor necrosis factor inhibitor therapy and risk of serious postoperative orthopedic infection in Rheumatoid Arthritis. Arthritis Care Res 2006;55:333–7.

18. Goodman SM, Springer B, Guyatt G, et al. 2017 American College of Rheumatology/American Association of Hip and Knee Surgeons guideline for the perioperative management of antirheumatic medication in patients with rheumatic diseases undergoing elective total hip or total knee arthroplasty. J Arthroplasty 2017;32(9):2628–38.

19. Amadio PC. Fungal infections of the hand. Hand Clin 1998;14(4):605–12.

20. Murray PM. Septic arthritis of the hand and wrist. Hand Clin 1998;14(4):579–87.

21. Dastagir K, Luketina R, Kuhbier JW, et al. Impact of delayed presentation of patients with hand infections to hand surgeons: a retrospective single-centre study of 379 patients. Handchir Mikrochir Plast Chir 2019;51(1):45–8.

22. Honda H, McDonald JR. Current recommendations in the management of osteomyelitis of the hand and wrist. J Hand Surg Am 2009;34(6):1135–6.

23. Reilly KE, Linz JC, Stern PJ, et al. Osteomyelitis of the tubular bones of the hand. J Hand Surg Am 1997;22(4):644–9.

24. Johnston BL, Conly JM. Osteomyelitis management: more art than science? Can J Infect Dis Med Microbiol 2007;18(2):115–8.

25. Mackowiak PA, Jones SR, Smith JW. Diagnostic value of sinus-tract cultures in chronic osteomyelitis. JAMA 1978;239(26):2772–5.

26. Pinder R, Barlow G. Osteomyelitis of the hand. J Hand Surg Eur Vol 2016;41(4):431–40.

27. Darouiche RO. Treatment of infections associated with surgical implants. N Engl J Med 2004;350(14): 1422–9.

28. Hara A, Yokoyama M, Ichihara S, et al. Masquelet technique for the treatment of acute osteomyelitis of the PIP joint caused by clenched-fist human bite injury: a case report. Int J Surg Case Rep 2018;51: 282–7.

29. Aimé VL, Kidwell JT, Webb LH. Single-stage treatment of osteomyelitis for digital salvage by using an antibiotic-eluting, methylmethacrylate joint-spanning spacer. J Hand Surg Am 2017;42(6): 480-.e1.

30. Draeger RW, Bynum DK Jr. Flexor tendon sheath infections of the hand. J Am Acad Orthop Surg 2012; 20(6):373–82.

31. Boles SD, Schmidt CC. Pyogenic flexor tenosynovitis. Hand Clin 1998;14(4):567–78.

32. Basadre JO, Parry SW. Indications for surgical debridement in 125 human bites to the hand. Arch Surg 1991;126(1):65–7.

33. Rizzo M. The use of Integra in hand and upper extremity surgery. J Hand Surg Am 2012;37(3):583–6.

34. Reynolds M, Kelly DA, Walker NJ, et al. Use of Integra in the management of complex hand wounds from cancer resection and nonburn trauma. Hand 2018;13(1):74–9.

Soft Tissue Coverage for Severe Infections

Vanessa Prokuski, MD[a,b], Adam Strohl, MD[c,*]

KEYWORDS

• Infection • Wound • Coverage • Debridement • Flap

KEY POINTS

- The most critical part of the treatment of a severe upper extremity infection is thorough debridement of involved tissues.
- Inability to clear infection or heal wounds is caused by many factors, such as immunocompromise, malnutrition, vascular insufficiency, and foreign bodies. Patients with these issues should be medically and nutritionally optimized to facilitate their healing; hyperbaric oxygen and negative pressure wound therapy are modalities that may aid in this.
- The decision on how to approach soft tissue coverage of upper extremity defects after infection is complex and requires consideration of the character and location of the wound, patient factors and desires, the anticipated functional results of the reconstruction, surgeon experience, and more.

INTRODUCTION

Upper extremity infections are a common ailment. Severe infections that require extensive debridement can cause soft tissue defects that have the potential to become difficult, clinical challenges for providers. An understanding of principles of management for clearing infection and coverage of any resultant wounds is essential for upper extremity surgeons. These principles include determining the infective organism and obtaining source control, determining appropriate coverage of soft tissue defects, and optimizing healing.

DISCUSSION
Setting the Stage

Evaluation of upper extremity infection

In evaluating a patient with a suspected upper extremity infection, a thorough history should be taken to obtain a complete picture of the ailment. Information should be obtained about causative factors (eg, trauma); quality and duration of symptoms; systemic symptoms, such as fever; previous treatment; recent illness; and immune status of the patient.[1] On examination, infections of the upper extremity often present with erythema, tenderness, and fluctuance. A wound or drainage may be present (**Fig. 1**). Proximal streaking of erythema or axillary lymphadenopathy indicate lymphangitic spread of infection.[1,2]

White blood cell count, C-reactive protein, and erythrocyte sedimentation rate should be obtained. In patients with severe infection or systemic illness, blood cultures should be taken.[2]

Imaging is helpful in evaluating some upper extremity infections if the diagnosis is not clear on clinical examination. Radiographs are the first-line imaging modality and can identify foreign bodies, such as needles; soft tissue swelling or gas; and evidence of osteomyelitis, such as loss of medullary trabeculae, focal cortical loss, and periosteal reaction. Ultrasound demonstrates fluid collections and can differentiate solid from cystic lesions, such as abscesses. It can also show a

[a] Philadelphia Hand to Shoulder Center/Jefferson, Philadelphia, PA, USA; [b] Orthopedic Care Physicians Network, 675 Paramount Drive, Suite 205, Raynham, MA 02767, USA; [c] Plastic and Reconstructive Surgery, Philadelphia Hand to Shoulder Center, Thomas Jefferson University Hospital, 834 Chestnut Street, Suite G-114, Philadelphia, PA 19107, USA
* Corresponding author.
E-mail address: ABStrohl@handcenters.com

Hand Clin 36 (2020) 369–379
https://doi.org/10.1016/j.hcl.2020.03.011

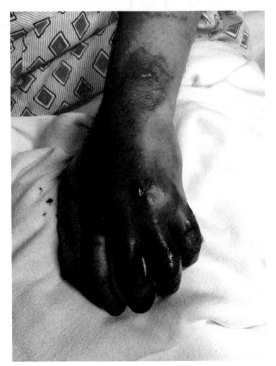

Fig. 1. Grossly swollen hand with areas of erythema, ulceration, and visible purulence.

"cobblestone" appearance of subcutaneous tissue caused by accumulation of edema; this is present in cellulitis, necrotizing fasciitis, and other infections. MRI is helpful in diagnosing soft tissue infection and can show thickening of subcutaneous tissues in cellulitis, focal lesions with high signal intensity with peripheral enhancement on administration of contrast in abscesses, joint effusion with synovitis in septic arthritis, fluid within the tendon sheath in infective tenosynovitis, and thickening of fascial planes with tracking fluid in necrotizing fasciitis.[3–7] In addition, MRI can demonstrate evidence of osteomyelitis, such as bone marrow edema, intraosseous and subperiosteal abscesses, and periostitis.[8] Computer tomography (CT) is limited by poorer soft tissue resolution than MRI, but is more widely available and generally quicker to obtain. CT can demonstrate subcutaneous emphysema in necrotizing fasciitis and contrast CT may yield rim-enhancing thick-walled fluid collection in abscesses. Multiple nuclear medicine studies exist and may be useful for patients in whom CT and MRI are contraindicated, but are often limited by low spatial resolution and availability.[6]

Several conditions can mimic upper extremity infections, such as gout, calcific tendinitis, and malignancy. Clinical examination and a positive response to nonsteroidal anti-inflammatory drugs may help distinguish an inflammatory condition from an infective one.[2] A mass, discoloration, tenderness, and ulceration are features that are found in infections and malignancies.[9] If a patient's lesion is firm, painful, and fixed in place, or if the patient describes systemic symptoms, such as weight loss or fatigue, the examiner should consider malignancy in the differential diagnosis.[1] Further evaluation of lesions concerning for malignancy includes laboratory studies (white blood cell count, C-reactive protein, erythrocyte sedimentation rate, chemistries, alkaline phosphatase) and imaging.[2] Radiographs can evaluate for bony abnormality that could indicate neoplasm and MRI can delineate the lesion's heterogeneity, location, size, and relationship to nearby structures.[9]

Treatment of upper extremity infection

Treatment of upper extremity infections is operative or nonoperative depending on the circumstance. In nonsuppuritic infections, such as uncomplicated cellulitis, patients may be treated with antibiotics and monitored closely.[10–12] However, in infections that involve a collection of purulent fluid, drainage is generally required.[2,10,11] The penetration of an antibiotic into an encapsulated collection of purulent fluid varies based on the antibiotic, organism, and maturity of the abscess. Even when a functional concentration of antibiotic is present within an abscess, multiple factors, such as low pH, antibiotic-deactivating enzymes, low oxygen tension, and high bacterial count, are postulated to render these medications ineffective, necessitating surgical intervention for abscess resolution.[13]

Debridement

Debridement of an infected wound is the most crucial part of treatment of a suppurative infection and later coverage.[14,15] Debridement of infection follows some general surgical principles. Incisions should be made large and should attempt to minimize exposure of tendons and neurovascular structures whenever possible, because the incision is generally left open. Extensive debridement of all infected and necrotic tissues including the abscess capsule is necessary to prevent recurrent infection. Contaminated or necrotic tissues are a primary reason for failure of flap coverage of upper extremity wounds[14,16] and if present extensive wound debridement should be performed until only uninfected, viable tissue remains. The mantra "all but the white stuff, unless necessary" highlights the extent of debridement goals while attempting to spare critical structures (tendons, nerves, bones) unless clearly involved (**Fig. 2**).

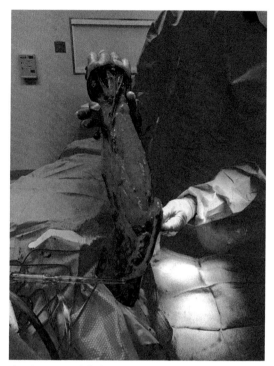

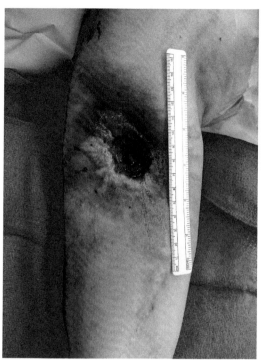

Fig. 2. Large, full-thickness wound of the upper extremity following multiple, sharp debridements for necrotizing fasciitis. Note the importance of exposed structures including tendons and bone.

Fig. 3. Predebridement. Chronic wound of the upper arm with communication to necrotic bone of the humerus. Note the induration and erythema of the surrounding soft tissues.

Remaining tissue must maintain an active blood supply or it will necrose and become a nidus for infection. It is recommended that initial debridement occur under tourniquet control to best identify and remove infected and devitalized tissue. Once this is accomplished the tourniquet is let down and tissue inspected for bleeding. If a portion of the wound does not have bleeding tissue, it likely has a compromised blood supply and should be debrided back until bleeding tissue is encountered.[14,16,17] Specimens for Gram stain and culture are obtained from the debrided tissue. If there is any question as to the possibility of a malignancy, specimens should be sent to pathology for evaluation. Once debridement is complete, extensive irrigation is performed. Wounds are left open or loosely approximated with a gauze wick in place to facilitate drainage of contaminated fluid.[2,11] It is sometimes difficult to assess the extent of tissue involvement in serious infections, so in these cases serial debridement is recommended to assist in the removal of all devitalized tissue. Debridement is performed every 2 to 3 days until the wound has clean, viable edges and base.[18] In severe cases, serial debridement may not be enough to control infection and amputation may be necessary (**Figs. 3 and 4**).[2]

Antibiotics

In most situations, antibiotics should be held until wound cultures are obtained to ensure that their administration does not erroneously affect the results of the culture. However, in cases of severe upper extremity infection with systemic illness the patient should receive immediate empiric antibiotic therapy with urgent surgical intervention as determined by the clinical picture.[2] Management of antibiotics is facilitated by an infectious diseases specialist who can determine the optimal combination of antibiotics by considering the most commonly encountered bacteria in the type of infection being treated and regional bacterial susceptibility patterns.[10] For instance, marine injuries, human or animal bites, and exposure to soil may warrant the addition of specific antibiotics.[2] Methicillin-resistant *Staphylococcus aureus* is the most common bacteria associated with hand infections, so empiric therapy typically includes vancomycin or other medications that remain active against this organism.[2,19–21] As culture and sensitivity data are available, antibiotics are tailored to the causative organism.[10]

Poor wound healing and refractory infection

Eradication of infection may be difficult in certain patients. Immunocompromised patients are at

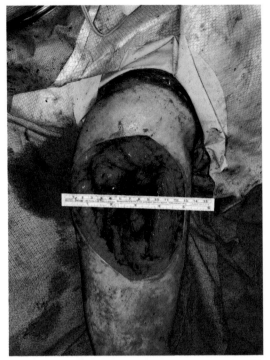

Fig. 4. Postdebridement. Upper arm wound with wide excision of soft tissues surrounding chronic wound and bone. Now, the wound is larger with more exposed structures including muscle, fascia, nerve, and bone.

risk for persistent infection, increased complication rates, and worse outcomes than other patients. Patients with immunocompromise include those with human immunodeficiency virus, diabetes, and autoimmune diseases; smokers; and individuals on immunosuppressants, such as patients receiving tumor necrosis factor-α inhibitors for various diseases.[1] In addition, malignancy can predispose patients to refractory infections; this is caused by cytotoxicity of chemotherapeutic agents or by immunodysfunction or obstructive processes stemming from the malignancy itself.[22] In immunocompromised patients, it is essential to

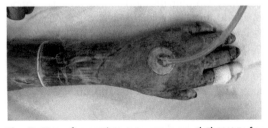

Fig. 5. Use of negative pressure wound therapy for the hand, using a sterile, surgical glove for help is maintaining adequate "air seal" in the web spaces.

use a multispecialty approach to optimize treatment of these conditions and facilitate infection control.

Malnutrition can also prevent wound healing and clearance of infections. Nearly all nutrient deficiencies can impair the normal immune response if the deficiency is severe enough. Most nutrients are involved in the process of protein synthesis, and most immune responses are protein-mediated. A disturbance in the creation of proteins used in immune responses may hamper the function of antibodies, reduce immunoglobulin concentrations, decrease lymphocyte count, reduce complement formation, cause dysfunction of T cells, and leave the body susceptible to infection. In addition, nutrient deficiency hinders the normal functioning of nonimmunologic defense systems of the body, such as the anatomic barriers of skin and mucosa, secretions of mucus and gastric acid, the gut microbiota, and the febrile response.[5] In patients with a nonhealing wound or refractory infection, a malnutrition work-up should be performed. This includes identification of patients with previous gastric bypass surgery, low body mass index, and malabsorptive and hypermetabolic states, which all may predispose to nutrient deficiency. Obese patients are also at risk for malnutrition, because high-calorie diets are often low on nutrients and high on fat and carbohydrates. Patients with cirrhosis and other liver diseases have poor protein synthesis, hematologic derangement, and often significant edema secondary to low oncotic pressure, even anasarca. Examination of at-risk patients includes evaluation of nails, hair, and skin turgor. Complete blood count with differential, reticulocyte count, serum albumin, prealbumin, serum transferrin, hemoglobin A_{1C}, and vitamin D levels should be checked. Patients should be optimized with the assistance of a nutritionist with input from other specialists, such as hematologists, depending on laboratory results[23]

Wounds after debridement of infection are treated with negative pressure wound therapy (NPWT) to facilitate healing (**Fig. 5**). NPWT uses a vacuum, which applies subatmospheric pressure to wounds.[24,25] This modality is used to protect a wound, ready it for coverage or closure, or create a viable bed for split-thickness skin grafts.[26] The application itself can deform and reduce wounds with repeated applications leading to eventual closure by aided secondary intention. It has been found to cause a four-fold increase in blood flow, significantly increase rate of granulation tissue formation, and diminish wound bacterial counts and the amount of collagen-degrading matrix metalloproteinases present.[24,26,27] NPWT cannot be used over exposed neurovascular structures, visceral organs, or eschar overlying necrotic tissue; use over exposed tendon or bone is controversial.[26] NPWT is used to facilitate formation of a layer of granulation tissue over various structures in a delayed, controlled fashion, while other patient factors are addressed appropriately.

Hyperbaric oxygen therapy (HBO) is used to treat wounds with delayed healing or persistent infection. This modality involves the administration of pure oxygen to patients in a pressurized chamber, which increases the oxygen content of the blood. HBO allows oxygen to reach the body's more hypoxic tissues and facilitates the diffusion of oxygen over greater distances. This improves wound healing by facilitating neovascularization and increasing growth factor production. Increased oxygen may also play an antimicrobial role in infected wounds, particularly when the pathogen is an anaerobe.[28] There are experimental data that suggest that HBO can promote healing of various tissues, such as bone[29] and nerves.[30] Studies have credited HBO with improving outcomes in mutilating hand injuries by combating tissue hypoxia and hastening healing.[31] In addition, it has been credited with facilitating the healing of diabetic hand infections.[32] Nonhealing wounds or wounds with refractory infection may benefit from HBO.

In a nonhealing wound, serial quantitative cultures are considered to attempt to determine whether there is a lingering infection preventing healing. The surface of a wound is not sterile and it is difficult to determine whether bacterial growth represents benign subclinical colonization or a clinically significant bacterial burden; this is the goal of quantitative cultures. The technique may yield useful information, but it has largely fallen out of favor with several studies suggesting that the correlation of culture findings to infection was unacceptably low.[33]

Coverage of Soft Tissue Defects Caused by Infection

Coverage decision making
Debridement of an infected wound may leave the upper extremity with a large soft tissue defect, which can prove challenging to cover definitely. An understanding of coverage options facilitates treatment of patients with these wounds. Coverage decisions must be made taking into account the wound location and size, exposure of critical structures, condition of surrounding tissues, injury complexity, and patient comorbidities.[34] In reconstructing hand and arm wounds, the primary principles of coverage are to restore

function, preserve sensibility and mobility, and strive to match the donor tissue with the tissue of the defect.[17]

Timing of coverage
Early studies suggested that soft tissue defects should be covered as soon as possible to prevent infection and flap failure.[14,29] Authors posited that wound fibrosis hampers attempts at microvascular reconstruction.[14] However, subsequent investigations have indicated that delayed coverage is safe and efficacious, with multiple studies demonstrating no difference in free flap outcome based on timing of reconstruction.[35,36] Some authors suggested that delayed coverage actually had a positive effect on flap outcomes, likely caused by the effect of multiple debridements.[37] NPWT is used in between debridements to minimize the bacterial count of the wound and optimize the wound bed for eventual coverage while finalizing soft tissue coverage plans.[17,24,35] In general, soft tissue reconstruction should occur as soon as possible once the wound is free from infection and devitalized tissue. Signs of infection clearance include resolution of edema and induration, positive skin wrinkles, lack of purulent drainage, and appearance of granulation tissue.[38] Efforts should be made to prevent desiccation of exposed structures, such as tendon, vessel, nerve, and/or bone.

The reconstructive ladder
The reconstructive ladder (**Fig. 6**) is a classic wound coverage concept wherein the simplest procedure to address a coverage issue is considered before moving up a rung to a more complicated procedure.[27,39] This progression typically starts with closure by secondary intention (although in some authors' ladders, direct closure is the first rung), then direct closure, regional flaps, and distant flaps[15,27]:

- Closure by secondary intention: The wound is left open and allowed to heal itself from inside out without any attempt to approximate the wound edges. This is helpful in infected wounds, because the incision is open and able to drain contaminated fluid freely.
- Direct, or primary, closure: The wound edges are opposed, ideally with minimal tension, with sutures, staples, and/or other methods and microscopically sealed within 24 hours.
- Skin grafting: This requires a well-vascularized wound bed with granulation tissue to "take" or be successful.[15] They are useful when the defect does not require any restoration of volume.[17] In defects caused by infection status post multiple

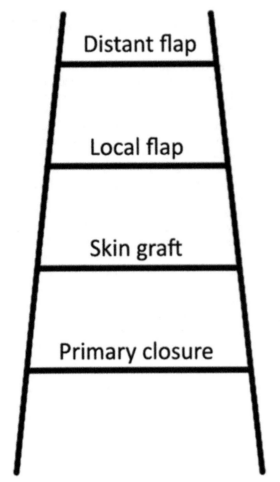

Fig. 6. The reconstructive ladder illustrating the traditional concept that the surgeon should begin with the less complex, lower rungs before moving on to the higher rungs in addressing soft tissue coverage. (*From* Janis JE, Kwon RK, Attinger CE. The new reconstructive ladder: modifications to the traditional model. Plast Reconstr Surg 2011;127(Suppl.):206S; with permission.)

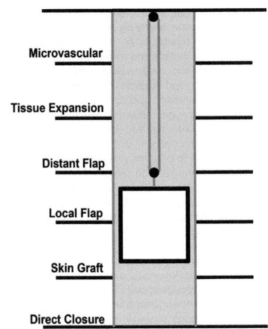

Fig. 7. The reconstructive elevator illustrating the newer concept that the surgeon can choose to move directly to a "higher" and more complex procedure if deemed necessary for the wound. (*From* Janis JE, Kwon RK, Attinger CE. The new reconstructive ladder: modifications to the traditional model. Plast Reconstr Surg. 2011;127 Suppl 1:205S–212S; with permission.)

debridements, it is possible that the wound bed may feature exposed bone without periosteum or tendon without peritenon, or be devoid of sufficient vasculature, which could preclude skin grafting alone. For larger areas, split-thickness skin grafts are more common, whereas full-thickness skin grafts are ideal around mobile joints, for various reasons beyond the scope of this article.

- Local flaps: These are for wounds with exposed neurovascular structures, exposed bone without periosteum, and wounds without enough vascularity to support skin grafts. These include rotational flaps, which can cover a wound with vascularized tissue

advancement flaps, cross-finger flaps, and island flaps for small hand wounds.[34] In situations of severe infection after multiple debridements, it is possible to have significant tissue loss with suboptimal surrounding tissue secondary to induration, contracture, and additional incisions. Consideration of local flaps for coverage must take into account the quality of surrounding tissue and its suitability for local transfer while maintaining its vascularity.

- Regional flaps: When local or adjacent tissues are insufficient, tissues from further distances are transposed to resurface wounds. For wounds of the upper extremity, these include the reverse lateral arm flap for distal wounds and the radial forearm flap for proximal wounds.
- Distant flaps: Vascularized tissue for wound coverage may need to be transferred from the torso, lower extremity, or other upper extremity. These flaps may be pedicled, such as the groin flap, requiring a second procedure to divide and inset the flap.
- Free tissue transfer: A composite flap of skin, fat, fascia, muscle, and/or bone is elevated on

a vascular pedicle from elsewhere in the body, which requires microsurgical anastomosis of artery and vein at the recipient site. Surgeons must be facile at microvascular procedures and ensure the recipient vessels have remained unharmed by infection and/or debridement.

The reconstructive elevator and other modifications

Other authors have taken issue with this coverage directive, suggesting perhaps a reconstructive "elevator" is a better model for treating coverage issues than the concept of a ladder (**Fig. 7**). In this schema, consideration of reconstructive options does not need to progress in a step-wise fashion. Instead, consideration of coverage can proceed based on what would provide the most functional and cosmetic outcome. The reconstructive elevator concept is based on the premise that the simplest solution is not necessarily the best solution.[17,40] For example, a substantial first web space wound may be more simply reconstructed with a skin graft, but postoperatively contracture of the scar may cause an adduction contracture of the thumb.[17] Those opposed to the step-wise coverage recommended by the reconstructive ladder believe that it does not take into account the many considerations that go into determining the optimal plan, which include the patient's condition and willingness to accept wound care, the nature of the wound, the anticipated functional results of the reconstruction, surgeon experience, the staff and facility available for the procedure and rehabilitation, and more.[27]

Some authors have reinvented the reconstructive ladder with newer wound coverage modalities. NPWT and dermal matrices are two such entities that do not fit neatly into the previous ladder concept but have achieved widespread clinical usage.[27]

NPWT can help build a layer of granulation tissue over structures that would have precluded immediate skin grafting, such as tendon or bone. Once there is sufficient tissue present over the critical structures, closure may then proceed with either skin grafting or healing by secondary intention.[27,41] It is used to facilitate any other type of coverage.[27] It is typically used to aid on coverage of smaller regions with exposed bone or tendon. It is not known what the largest surface area is that NPWT can treat, although one prospective study found that foot and ankle wounds up to 150 cm^2 were able to be successfully treated with NPWT and subsequent skin grafting.[42] The area that NPWT is able to successfully help cover is likely to be determined by patient factors and the proportion of exposed tissue comprised of bone or other nongraftable structures. In addition to sequential application of NPWT and skin grafting, NPWT has also been described as a concomitant adjunct to skin grafting to improve graft incorporation and minimize complications, such as seroma beyond the graft and shearing.[41]

Some authors believe that acellular dermal matrices and regenerative wound matrices deserve a place in the reconstructive ladder schema.[27] Dermal matrices are soft connective tissue grafts made of decellularized skin from humans, pigs, or other species and composed primarily of collagen and chondroitin-6-sulfate. Other regenerative wound matrices are engineered with similar structures. They act as a scaffold to support vascular ingrowth from the underlying wound bed over the course of weeks.[27,43] Once matured, these matrices are almost always covered by skin grafts. When used with skin grafting, the resultant skin is thicker, more elastic, less prone to contraction, and more like native skin than when split-thickness skin grafting is used alone.[27] Like NPTW, these matrices are used to cover tissues that are not able to be directly covered by skin grafts, such as bone, tendon, and cartilage.[27] Authors recommend that once the matrix develops a

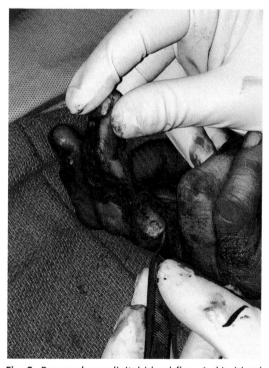

Fig. 8. Reverse homodigital island flap. A skin island based on retrograde flow through the underlying digital artery is dissected and ready to be transposed 180-degrees to the fingertip pulp.

peach color, it is fully vascularized and can support skin grafting; this may take 2 to 4 weeks.[44] These matrices are used to cover large areas, unlike NPWT, which is typically reserved for smaller discrete regions requiring coverage.[27] They are not appropriate for situations in which there is inadequate vasculature of the wound bed or in lingering infection[45] because they are technically foreign bodies. Additionally, one must consider the cost of such products and their ultimate place in the reconstructive toolbox for covering soft tissue defects.

Types of Flaps

For each type of flap, there are many different examples. Availability of tissues, patient factors, and familiarity of the surgeon dictate selection of individual flaps. The extent of different flaps is beyond the scope of this article, but some of the more commonly used flaps are reviewed next.

Local flaps and regional flaps

- Homodigital island flap: For coverage of small defects on the volar and dorsal fingers less than ~2.5 × 3 cm.[17] This axial-pattern flap entails dissection of the digital artery from the nerve, and is based anterograde or retrograde. The donor site requires skin grafting (**Fig. 8**).
- Cross-finger Flap: For volar defects less than 2 cm on the digit. It entails creation of a random pattern flap from the dorsal surface of the middle or proximal phalanx that is flipped from a neighboring finger to the defect of the affected finger and allowed to remain there until the donor site has incorporated it. The donor site requires a skin graft. The reverse cross-finger is designed for covering dorsal wounds and uses only an adipofascial flap and skin graft on the wounded finger. The second procedure is typically performed 2 weeks later to divide and inset the flap from the donor digit. Stiffness of the involved digits is possible postoperatively.[17,46]
- First dorsal metacarpal artery flap: This flap may be used to cover defects of the thumb 5 cm in length by 3 cm in width.[17] A branch of the dorsal radial sensory nerve is included in flap dissection to allow for a sensate flap coverage. The donor site overlying the index proximal phalanx requires skin graft coverage.
- Posterior interosseous artery flap: Designed to be based on retrograde flow through the anterior interosseous artery just proximal to the wrist, this flap can cover significant dorsal hand and digital wounds. The donor site of the

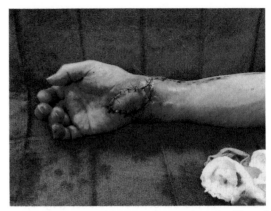

Fig. 9. Reverse radial forearm flap. A skin island based on retrograde flow through the underlying radial artery has been transposed from the radial border of the mid-forearm to cover a palmar wound distally.

proximal, dorsal forearm typically requires skin grafting for secondary donor coverage.
- Radial forearm flap: Based on the radial artery, its vena comitantes, and sometimes the cephalic vein, this is rotated to cover elbow and antecubital wounds. When the donor

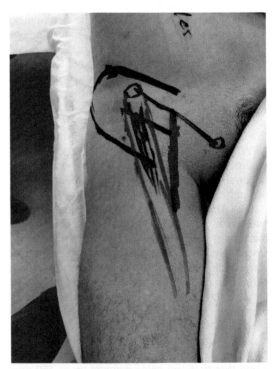

Fig. 10. Traditional markings for a groin flap before harvest. Iliac/femoral artery (*red*), sartorius muscle (*green*), inguinal ligament (*black*), proposed incision for medially based flap (*blue*; *central line* is superficial circumflex iliac artery).

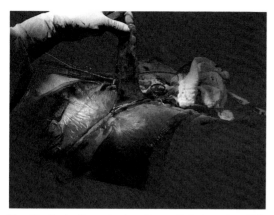

Fig. 11. Groin flap raised on its medially based pedicle of the superficial circumflex iliac artery with lateral donor site primarily closed and now ready to be sewn to the upper extremity soft tissue defect.

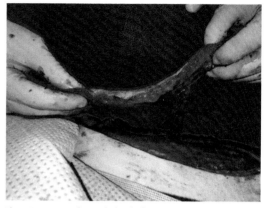

Fig. 13. Anterolateral thigh flap. Fasciocutaneous flap based on perforators (seen below the subcutaneous tissues) emanating from the descending branch of the lateral circumflex femoral artery.

skin paddle is designed over the proximal forearm, it is rotated distally to cover dorsal or volar wounds through retrograde flow in the radial artery. Its donor site typically requires skin grafting (**Fig. 9**).

Distant flaps: pedicled

- Groin flap: This axial flap based on the superficial circumflex iliac artery allows harvest of tissue up to 25 cm long and 10 cm wide. This flap requires the recipient site to be secured to the donor site at the groin for 3 weeks.[17] Hygiene is difficult during immobilization and shoulder/elbow stiffness can result from the immobilization (**Figs. 10–12**).
- Thoracoabdominal flap: This flap is large and is based on the epigastric artery with

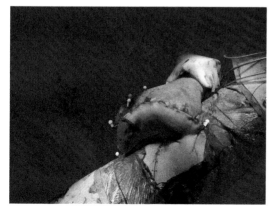

Fig. 12. Groin flap sewn to a hand defect for coverage of multiple, exposed metacarpal bones. Note the similar color of flap skin to surrounding areas without evidence of congestion or ischemia.

similarities to the previously described groin flap.

Distant flaps: free

- Lateral arm flap: A portion of skin and subcutaneous tissue 15 cm in length and 6 cm in width based on the posterior radial collateral artery may be harvested to provide coverage for a more distal soft tissue defect. Its anatomy is similar to the reverse lateral arm flap that is used as a pedicled flap for elbow defects.[17]
- Radial forearm flap: Similar to the previously described pedicled regional flap, this flap is based on the length of the radial artery and accompanied by the cephalic vein.
- Anterolateral thigh flap: This workhorse flap based on perforators from the lateral circumflex femoral artery from the thigh allows transfer of a tissue island up to 22 cm long and 9 cm wide, or larger if skin grafted (**Fig. 13**). Its deep facial surface can provide a superior gliding surface, which is ideal for tendon repairs or extensor tendons. It is thick and may require future debulking procedures for optimal cosmesis. Harvesting a suprafascial anterolateral thigh flap may minimize undesirable flap thickness.[17]

SUMMARY

Coverage of soft tissue defects in the upper extremity caused by infection and debridement of infected tissue is a challenging problem. Treatment starts with prompt identification and eradication of infection, including antibiotics and extensive debridement. Optimizing the patient's medical and nutritional status can facilitate eradication of infection and wound healing. Coverage of soft tissue defects caused by infection and debridement demands consideration of many factors. Options include healing by primary or secondary intention, skin grafts, local flaps, and distant flaps. NPWT and acellular dermal matrices can also aid in coverage.

DISCLOSURE

A. Strohl is a stockholder for PolarityTE (not mentioned nor referred to in this article).

REFERENCES

1. Teo WZW, Chung KC. Hand infections. Clin Plast Surg 2019;46:371–81.
2. Wolfe S, Pederson W, Kozin S, et al. Green's operative hand surgery. 7th edition. Philadelphia: Elsevier; 2016.
3. Chang CD, Wu JS. Imaging of musculoskeletal soft tissue infection. Semin Roentgenol 2017;52(1):55–62.
4. Palestro CJ, Charito L, Miller TT. Imaging of musculoskeletal infections. Best Pract Res Clin Rheumatol 2006;20:1197–218.
5. Scrimshaw NS, SanGiovanni JP. Synergism of nutrition, infection, and immunity: an overview. Am J Clin Nutr 1997;66:464S–77S.
6. Turecki MB, Taljanovic MS, Stubbs AY, et al. Imaging of musculoskeletal soft tissue infections. Skeletal Radiol 2010;39:957–71.
7. Wang HD, Alonso-Escalante JC, Cho BH, et al. Versatility of free cutaneous flaps for upper extremity soft tissue reconstruction. J Hand Microsurg 2017;9: 058–66.
8. Lee YJ, Sadigh S, Mankad K, et al. The imaging of osteomyelitis. Quant Imaging Med Surg 2016;6:184.
9. Henderson MM, Neumeister MW, Bueno RA Jr. Hand tumors: I. skin and soft-tissue tumors of the hand. Plast Reconstr Surg 2014;133:154e–64e.
10. Chahine EB, Sucher AJ. Skin and soft tissue infections. PSAP 2015;1:1–27.
11. Henry M. Hand infections. Curr Orthop Pract 2018; 29:105–9.
12. Jackson KA, Bohm MK, Brooks JT, et al. Invasive methicillin-resistant Staphylococcus aureus infections among persons who inject drugs—six sites, 2005–2016. Morb Mortal Wkly Rep 2018;67:625.
13. Bamberger DM. Outcome of medical treatment of bacterial abscesses without therapeutic drainage: review of cases reported in the literature. Clin Infect Dis 1996;23:592–603.
14. Godina M. Early microsurgical reconstruction of complex trauma of the extremities. Orthop Trauma Dir 2006;4:29–35.
15. Scott LL. The reconstructive ladder. Tech Orthop 1995;10:88–93.
16. Lister G, Luis S. Emergency free flaps to the upper extremity. J Hand Surg 1988;13:22–8.
17. Miller EA, Friedrich J. Soft tissue coverage of the hand and upper extremity: the reconstructive elevator. J Hand Surg 2016;41:782–92.
18. Chen SH, Wei FC, Chen HC, et al. Emergency free-flap transfer for reconstruction of acute complex extremity wounds. Plast Reconstr Surg 1992;89:882–8.
19. Koshy JC, Bell B. Hand infections. J Hand Surg 2019;44(1):46–54.
20. Kourtis AP, Hatfield K, Baggs J, et al. Vital signs: epidemiology and recent trends in methicillin-resistant and in methicillin-susceptible Staphylococcus aureus bloodstream infections—United States. Morb Mortal Wkly Rep 2019;68:214.
21. McDonald LS, Bavaro MF, Hofmeister EP, et al. Hand infections. J Hand Surg 2011;36:1403–12.
22. Kofteridis DP, Valachis A, Koutsounaki E, et al. Skin and soft tissue infections in patients with solid tumours. ScientificWorldJ 2012;2012:804518.
23. Golladay GJ, Jibananda S, Jiranek WA. Patient optimization—strategies that work: malnutrition. J Arthroplasty 2016;31:1631–4.
24. Desai KK, Hahn E, Pulikkottil B, et al. Negative pressure wound therapy: an algorithm. Clin Plast Surg 2012;39:311–24.
25. Downs DJ, Wongworawat MD, Gregorius SF. Timeliness of appropriate antibiotics in hand infections. Clin Orthop Relat Res 2007;461:17–9.
26. Lesiak AC, Shafritz AB. Negative-pressure wound therapy. J Hand Surg 2013;38:1828–32.
27. Janis JE, Kwon RK, Attinger CE. The new reconstructive ladder: modifications to the traditional model. Plast Reconstr Surg 2011;127:205S–12S.
28. Nassab PF. Understanding hyperbaric oxygen therapy and its role in the upper extremity. J Hand Surg 2011;36:529–31.
29. Chen WJ, Lai PL, Chang CH, et al. The effect of hyperbaric oxygen therapy on spinal fusion: using the model of posterolateral intertransverse fusion in rabbits. J Trauma Acute Care Surg 2002;52:333–8.
30. Eguiluz-Ordoñez R, Sánchez CE, Venegas A, et al. Effects of hyperbaric oxygen on peripheral nerves. Plast Reconstr Surg 2006;118:350–7.
31. Chiang IH, Yuan ST, Shun CC. Is hyperbaric oxygen therapy indispensable for saving mutilated hand injuries? Int Wound J 2017;14:929–36.
32. Aydin F, Kaya A, Savran A, et al. Diabetic hand infections and hyperbaric oxygen therapy. Acta Orthop Traumatol Turc 2014;48:649–54.
33. Kallstrom G. Are quantitative bacterial wound cultures useful? J Clin Microbiol 2014;52:2753–6.
34. Griffin M, Hindocha S, Malahias M, et al. Suppl 2: M3: flap decisions and options in soft tissue coverage of the upper limb. Open Orthop J 2014;8:409.

35. Gupta A, Lakhiani C, Lim BH, et al. Free tissue transfer to the traumatized upper extremity: risk factors for postoperative complications in 282 cases. J Plast Reconstr Aesthet Surg 2015;68:1184–90.

36. Steiert AE, Gohritz A, Schreiber TC, et al. Delayed flap coverage of open extremity fractures after previous vacuum-assisted closure (VAC) therapy–worse or worth? J Plast Reconstr Aesthet Surg 2009;62:675–83.

37. Yaremchuk MJ, Brumback RJ, Manson PN, et al. Acute and definitive management of traumatic osteocutaneous defects of the lower extremity. Plast Reconstr Surg 1987;80:1–14.

38. Woon CY, Lee JY, Teoh LC. Flap resurfacing of post-infection soft-tissue defects of the hand. Plast Reconstr Surg 2007;120:1922–9.

39. Simman R. Wound closure and the reconstructive ladder in plastic surgery. J Am Coll Certif Wound Spec 2009;1:6–11.

40. Gottlieb LJ, Krieger LM. From the reconstructive ladder to the reconstructive elevator. Plast Reconstr Surg 1994;93(7):1503–4.

41. Niimi Y, Ito H, Sakurai H. Negative-pressure wound therapy for fixing full-thickness skin graft on the thumb. JPRAS Open 2018;18:22–7.

42. Lee HJ, Kim JW, Oh CW, et al. Negative pressure wound therapy for soft tissue injuries around the foot and ankle. J Orthop Surg Res 2009;4:14.

43. Boháč M, Danišovič Ľ, Koller J, et al. What happens to an acellular dermal matrix after implantation in the human body? A histological and electron microscopic study. Eur J Histochem 2018;62:1.

44. Moiemen NS, Staiano JJ, Ojeh NO, et al. Reconstructive surgery with a dermal regeneration template: clinical and histologic study. Plast Reconstr Surg 2001;108:93–103.

45. Ellis CV, Kulber DA. Acellular dermal matrices in hand reconstruction. Plast Reconstr Surg 2012;130(5S-2):256S–69S.

46. Atasoy E. The reverse cross finger flap. J Hand Surg 2016;41:122–8.

Pediatric Hand Infections

Joseph F. Styron, MD, PhD

KEYWORDS

• Pediatric hand infection • Antibiotics • Paronychia • Thumb sucking • Seymour fracture

KEY POINTS

- Infections are an important source of morbidity in pediatric hands that come from frequent exposure to mouths and other dangers while exploring the world.
- Although *Staphylococcus aureus* is still the most common organism in pediatric hand infections, it is less common than in adults because pediatric patients are more likely to develop mixed aerobic/anaerobic infections or group A *Streptococcus pyogenes* infection.
- Pediatric patients with open physes potentially may sustain Seymour fractures of the distal phalanges that may become infected and sources for osteomyelitis if not recognized early.

INTRODUCTION

Considering the frequency with which children use their hands to explore the world, including their own mouths, mouths of other people, and mouths of animals, it is perhaps most surprising that children do not develop hand infections more frequently. The hand is the part of the body most frequently injured.[1] Fortunately, children rarely suffer from the same risk exposures that predispose adults to hand infections, such as diabetes or other systemic comorbidities, intravenous drug abuse, and hazardous work environments. Pediatric patients present unique challenges to treatment because a detailed history or chronology often is difficult to ascertain.

GENERAL ASSESSMENT

Whenever possible, the child or their caregiver should be questioned to determine the etiology and chronicity of the infection. Infections that may have started as superficial may progress to deep space infections due to an inability to recognize the developing infection in a more expedient manner. A history of trauma, recent illnesses or sick contacts, and environmental exposures is particularly important to discern. In addition, ascertaining the immunization status of the child is important as are any prior attempts at medical management, such as antibiotic prescriptions from another health care provider.

When examining an infected hand, the principles of examining an injury in the child should be kept in mind. Start by observing the child and how he/she is holding or using the extremity. Is he/she moving the shoulder, elbow, or wrist on his/her own? Often children become reflexively resistant to any movement of an arm due to apprehension, so, prior to laying hands on the child, try observing how he/she uses the arm and digits while left alone. Then start examining the extremity away from the obvious area of infection. Examine proximal joints through passive motion to evaluate for possible septic arthritis or proximal lymphadenitis. Finally, focus on the area of primary concern. Examine the hand for swelling. The dorsum of the hand frequently is edematous regardless of the actual location of infection due to the lymphatic drainage being most prominent there. The palmar aponeurosis provides a tighter connection between the skin and underlying structures; thus, the volar surface of the hand is less prone to pronounced swelling than the dorsal hand. The dorsum of the hand has been referred to as a red herring due to its propensity for swelling even if it is not the locus of infection.[2,3] When erythema is present, outlining the edges of the erythema with a skin marker is helpful for tracking progression versus regression over time.

9500 Euclid Avenue Mail Code A40, Cleveland, OH 44195, USA
E-mail address: styronj@ccf.org

Hand Clin 36 (2020) 381–386
https://doi.org/10.1016/j.hcl.2020.03.012

Imaging is helpful for a variety of reasons. Subcutaneous air visible on radiographs is concerning for gas gangrene whereas bony changes may be evidence of osteomyelitis. Ultrasound examination is a quick and inexpensive method to identify if any fluid collections are present. An abscess warrants a surgical decompression and débridement. Computed tomography and magnetic resonance imaging also can be helpful in identifying an underlying abscess or the presence of osteomyelitis.

Blood work should be ordered for almost all hand infections. Basic laboratory tests, such as a complete blood cell count with differential, as well as inflammatory markers for trending recovery, such as erythrocyte sedimentation rate and C-reactive protein, easily are obtained. Blood cultures along with wound cultures (if purulence is expressed, not just swabbing the skin surface) are extremely helpful for narrowing the spectrum of antibiotics. Unlike in adults in whom S aureus comprises between 50% and 80% of hand infections, in children, only 37% to 47% have S aureus as the primary organism.[4] Pediatric patients are more likely to have aerobic/anaerobic mixed infections (29%) and group A Streptococcus pyogenes infection (20%).[5,6] Swabbing under the fingernails to look for MRSA, particularly in children of health care workers, may help identify patients at increased risk for a methicillin-resistant S aureus

(MRSA) soft tissue infection.[7] A list of empiric antibiotic treatments is provided in **Table 1**.

In general, initial treatment of early infections can be resting the soft tissues with forearm-based splinting, elevation of the hand, and empiric antibiotic treatment (either oral or intravenous). Indications for surgical intervention include the presence of an abscess or systemic toxicity.

Children get the same types of hand infections as adults: paronychia, felons, flexor tenosynovitis, deep space infection, human and animal bite wounds, septic arthritis, and osteomyelitis. Each is described briefly in terms of presentation, etiology, and treatment strategies.

PARONYCHIA

Paronychia in pediatric patients, just like in adults, is an infection of the nail folds. The term typically is applied to infections of either the lateral nail folds (paronychium) or of the proximal nail fold (eponychium). It is manifested with localized pain, erythema, and swelling along the nail fold(s). Due to the frequent oral manipulation of their digits, paronychia in children differ from those in adults with mixed anaerobic and aerobic infectious organisms. As a result, broad-spectrum antibiotics, such as amoxicillin/clavulanate or clindamycin, is an appropriate initial treatment. The presence of purulence necessitates an incision and drainage,

Table 1
Common infecting organisms and antibiotic treatments

Type of Infection	Most Common Organism	Empiric Antibiotic Coverage
Acute paronychia	S aureus	Dicloxacillin
Chronic paronychia	Fungi	Topical corticosteroids and antifungals
Felon	S aureus	Dicloxacillin
Herpetic whitlow	Herpes simplex virus type 1 or type 2	Acyclovir
Pyogenic flexor tenosynovitis	S aureus	Vancomycin plus cefotaxime
Deep space infection	S aureus	Vancomycin plus ampicillin/sulbactam (Community acquired)
Human bite	S aureus and Eikenella corrodens	Superficial: amoxicillin/clavulanate; or deep: ampicillin/sulbactam
Animal bite	Gram-positive cocci and Pasteurella multocida	Superficial: amoxicillin/clavulanate; or deep: ampicillin/sulbactam
Septic arthritis	S aureus	Vancomycin plus efotaxime or ceftriaxone
Osteomyelitis	S aureus	Vancomycin plus cefotaxime or ceftriaxone (oral antibiotics are acceptable as well)

which is curative when coupled with antibiotics. If a child has been recently hospitalized, providing better MRSA coverage is warranted with vancomycin or linezolid; however, oral clindamycin and trimethoprim/sulfamethoxazole also may be used.[8,9] The surgical steps for addressing nail bed infections, such as paronychia, can be seen in **Box 1**.

Chronic paronychia are challenging to treat due to their polymicrobial etiology. They often are treated with topical creams that combine antifungals with steroids (3% clioquinol in triamcinolone-nystatin mixture). Occasionally, refractory cases of chronic paronychia may need to be treated with marsupialization with or without removal of the nail plate.

FELON

A pediatric felon is identical to that of adults in the sense that it a closed space infection of the fingertip pulp. Due to the multiple septae in the distal pulp, there are walled-off areas that, when inoculated, easily can develop into a localized abscess, causing pain, swelling, and erythema. If recognized early, a felon can be treated with antibiotics and rest, but felons present frequently after abscess formation, necessitating surgical intervention.[10] A high lateral incision followed by blunt dissection across all septae in the distal pulp to assure complete decompression of the abscess is the preferred technique. Placing the incision here avoids

---

> **Box 1**
> **Technique for paronychia infection**
>
> 1. A proximal digital block can be performed, with or without intravenous sedation, given a patient's age and cooperation.
>
> 2. A Freer elevator or another blunt instrument can be used to elevate the nail plate off, away from the affected nail fold.
>
> 3. If obvious purulent material is present beneath the nail plate, either a sliver of the nail plate may be sharply excised or the entire nail plate removed.
>
> 4. If the infection affects the eponychial fold, relaxing longitudinal incisions in the corners, in line with the paronychial folds, provides easier exposure by folding back the eponychium.
>
> 5. Once the wound is washed thoroughly, a small strip of gauze or the native nail plate may be gently placed back under the eponychial fold so that the nail matrix does not scar and close that space.

---

disruption of the volar fat pad or damage to the digital nerve and artery. In addition, consideration of which digit is involved dictates the preferred side of the nail to for the incision. Leaving a drain in place while administering empiric antibiotics and splinting the digit for immobilization may help expedite resolution of the infection. Debridement of the felon may be performed with a digital block with or without conscious sedation but alternatively may require general anesthesia depending on the age and maturity of the patient.

PYOGENIC FLEXOR TENOSYNOVITIS

It has been more than 100 years since Dr Allen Kanavel[11] first described his cardinal signs of flexor tenosynovitis: tenderness over the flexor tendons heath; finger held in a partially flexed posture; pain with passive extension; and uniform swelling of the entire finger. Although not all of Kanavel's signs typically are present, a suspicion of flexor tenosynovitis should warrant prompt treatment. His description of flexor tenosynovitis was built firmly on a thorough understanding of anatomy, in particular, how the bacterial infection can occupy the flexor tendon sheath between the distal interphalangeal joint and the A1 pulley. The dreaded horseshoe abscess can occur because the thumb flexor tendon sheath is continuous with the radial bursa while the small finger flexor tendon sheath is continuous with the ulna bursa and then there are communications between the radial and ulna bursae via Parona space.[10]

Developing infections detected early can be managed nonoperatively with splint immobilization, elevation, and antibiotics. Surgical débridement often is required, however, because many of these cases do not present until there are signs of fluctuance and certainly should be undertaken in the setting of systemic illness. Delay in surgical débridement may result in difficult complications, including tendon adhesions or even necrosis. Performing a full open approach versus a limited incision approach can be at the surgeon's discretion, depending on the severity of the infection and the surgeon's comfort level with the approach. If performing a full open exposure, midlateral exposure is preferable to Bruner incision to avoid necrosis of the skin flap tips. With a limited approach, using a 5-French pediatric feeding tube can assist with closed catheter irrigation.

DEEP SPACE INFECTIONS

There are multiple closed spaces within the hand, all of which can develop an abscess. These deep space infections often develop from extension of other infections or penetrating trauma but also rarely may develop from hematogenous spread of an infection. The segment of the hand involved determines the surgical approach to best access and decompress the infection. These spaces include the thenar space, space of Parona, interdigital subfascial spaces, and dorsal subaponeurotic space.

The dorsal subaponeurotic space is bounded by the extensor tendons dorsally and the metacarpals and interosseous muscles volarly. Abscesses here tend to be superficial, and longitudinal incisions to irrigate and débride the abscess should be centered over either the index metacarpal or between the fourth and fifth metacarpals but not directly over the extensor tendons.

The interdigital subfascial spaces are what become infected with a collar-button abscess. These infections are dumbbell-shaped, similar to old collar buttons, and often start volarly then spread peripherally dorsally but remain narrow in the middle. Surgical débridement can be performed by a volar incision with excision of the interdigital fascia, allowing the entire abscess to be drained. Incisions through the first web space should be avoided to minimize the chances of wound contractures limiting postoperative mobility. These wounds often are allowed to close via secondary intention.

Parona space may become infected via spread of infection from either the radial or ulna bursa. This manifests itself in pain with finger flexion and even acute carpal tunnel syndrome. Treatment of horseshoe abscesses is open surgical débridement while protecting the median nerve and flexor tendons.

The thenar space is bounded by the adductor pollicis dorsally, the index finger flexor tendon volarly, the adductor pollicis insertion on the proximal phalanx radially, and the midpalmar septum ulnarly. When this space is filled, the thumb tends to be held in a characteristic palmarly abducted position. A variety of incisions to decompress the thenar space have been defined and any of them may be used with the proviso that any incision running parallel to the commissure is discouraged to minimize the chances of a first web space contracture.

BITE WOUNDS
Human Bites

In younger children, bite wound injuries may be self-inflicted out of frustration or anger whereas in adolescents and young adults, a fight bite is the more common case. Due to the hand often being in a different position during the bite than it is

held during examination, careful examination must be taken to avoid missed pockets of infection. A saline load challenge may be performed of the finger joints to evaluate for communication between a joint and outside world. This may help decrease the changes of a potential missed, developing septic arthritis. Treatment of these human bites requires surgical drainage and irrigation along with débridement of the necrotic or nonviable tissue. Most providers perform open packing of the wound with healing allowed by secondary intention. Although S aureus remains the most common organism isolated in these injuries, Eikenella corrodens is a gram-negative rod frequently isolated in these human bite injuries. Why this is important to recall is because Eikenella corrodens is not sensitive to penicillinase-resistant penicillins or cephalosporins alone. Ampicilin/sulbactam is a great oral antibiotic option whereas children with penicillin allergies may be treated with trimethoprim/sulfamethoxazole.

Animal Bites

Children love animals and seem to love placing their hands in animals' mouths. More than half of annual dog bites in the United States involve children under the age of 12.[3] Knowing the animal that produced the bite also may help direct treatment strategies because cat bites tend to be more worrisome than dog bites. A dog's teeth tend to be less sharp and do most of their damage through a tearing motion that makes for ugly wounds with significant soft tissue damage, but the wound typically is larger and allows for drainage. A cat bite by contrast is more worrisome because a cat's teeth are like small infected hypodermic needles that can inoculate the deep tissue with bacteria, creating puncture wounds that quickly heal over, allowing the inoculated deep tissues to fester into an abscess. Although dog bites account for an overwhelming majority of animal bites overall (80%–90%), cat bites are responsible for a majority of animal bites that actually go on to develop infections (76%).[12] Management of animal bites is similar to that of human bites except additional consideration should be given for the unique organisms potentially present in the animal's saliva. Antibiotic coverage for Pasteurella multocida, Bacteroides, and Streptococcus viridans should be kept in mind when treating empirically. Penicillin is the preferred antibiotic for Pasteurella multocida.

SEPTIC ARTHRITIS

Direct inoculation is the most common cause of septic arthritis. This may occur from bite injuries

A   **B**

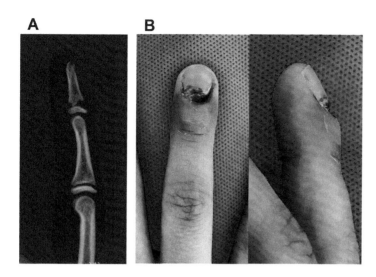

Fig. 1. (*A*) Radiograph of a Seymour fracture that was neglected by a 14-year-old patient for 1 month, believing he had just jammed his finger. (*B*) Clinical photo prior to decompression and removal of the nail plate to repair the nail bed. [*B*] (left) AP view; (right) lateral view with prominence noted of the proximal nail fold.

to the digits; otherwise, septic arthritis of the small joints of the fingers is quite rare. Larger joints, such as the wrist, elbow, and shoulder, are more likely to be affected. Upon examination, the swollen, erythematous joint is painful with any active or passive motion. A joint aspiration is necessary to confirm the diagnosis of a septic joint, looking at the fluid analysis' complete blood cell count with a differential and cultures of the fluid. Consensus for a white blood cell count (WBC) threshold for a diagnosis of septic arthritis does not exist but many experts loosely set the threshold at greater than 50,000 WBC/mm.[3] Surgical débridement of the joint typically is the treatment necessary for a septic arthritis.

A notable exception to surgical intervention is gonococcal arthritis, which is more common in women, and the wrist joint is the most commonly affected joint. If suspicious for a gonococcal infection, the aspirate should be grown on a chocolate agar (a specific request typically is required). The treatment of choice for gonococcal arthritis is penicillin; surgical intervention rarely is required for a gonococcal arthritis.

OSTEOMYELITIS

Osteomyelitis may affect the upper extremity of the pediatric patients. The most commonly affected areas of the upper extremity include the metaphyseal area of the proximal humerus, the distal radius, and the distal ulna, whereas the metacarpal is the most common area in the hand. A high index of suspicion and imaging helps determine the presence of underlying osteomyelitis. Laboratory tests often are misleadingly negative given the sequestered nature of the infection

within the bone. Fracture of the distal phalanx in which the nail bed becomes incarcerated in the now hinged open dorsal aspect of the physis can set the hand up for an open injury that often goes unrecognized, called a Seymour fracture. If unrecognized or untreated, a Seymour fracture may become infected and a source osteomyelitis (**Fig. 1**).[13]

In the absence of a focal fluid collection, initial management with prolonged antibiotics may be performed (4–6 weeks minimum or until symptom and sign resolution). Antibiotics may be administered intravenously or orally, depending on the susceptibility of the organism. Otherwise, in the setting of a Seymour fracture or formation of a focal fluid collection, treatment should consist of surgical débridement.

SUMMARY

Although many of the principles in management are the same in pediatric and adult patients, treating physicians should bear in mind the unique environments and characteristics of the pediatric hand when managing antibiotics and determining surgical intervention. Unique features of the pediatric hand help distinguish infections from their common counterparts in the adult hand, including the frequency of fingers in mouths from thumb sucking or nail biting, open growth plates, and typically more robust circulation with fewer systemic comorbidities. The infectious organism often is slightly different among pediatric patients compared with adults. Many of these infections can be managed with oral antibiotics unless a discrete collection of fluid, such as an abscess, has formed.

REFERENCES

1. Upton J, Littler JW, Eaton RG. Primary care of the injured hand, part 1. Postgrad Med 1979;66(2):115–20.
2. Carter PR. Hand infections. Philadelphia: Saunders Co. Ltd; 1983.
3. Kroonen L. Pediatric hand infections. In: Abzug J, Kozin SH, Zlotolow D, editors. The pediatric upper extremity. 1st edition. New York: Springer; 2015. p. 1301–22.
4. Abrams RA, Botte MJ. Hand infections: treatment recommendations for specific types. J Am Acad Orthop Surg 1996;4(4):219–30.
5. Fowler JR, Ilyas AM. Epidemiology of adult acute hand infections at an urban medical center. J Hand Surg Am 2013;38(6):1189–93.
6. Harness N, Blazar PE. Causative microorganisms in surgically treated pediatric hand infections. J Hand Surg Am 2005;30(6):1294–7.
7. Muschick KD, LaCroix R, McAdams J. Fingernail carriage of methicillin-resistant staphylococcus aureus and possible correlation with soft tissue infections in children. South Med J 2016;109(4):236–9.
8. Grome L, Borah G. Neonatal acute paronychia. Hand (N Y) 2017;12(5):NP99–100.
9. Shafritz AB, Coppage JM. Acute and chronic paronychia of the hand. J Am Acad Orthop Surg 2014;22(3):165–74.
10. McDonald LS, Bavaro MF, Hofmeister EP, et al. Hand infections. J Hand Surg Am 2011;36A:1403–12.
11. Kanavel AB. Infections of the hand: a guide to the surgical treatment of acute and chronic suppurative processes in the fingers, hand and forearm. Philadelphia: Lea & Febiger; 1912.
12. Teo WZW, Chung KC. Hand infections. Clin Plast Surg 2019;46(3):371–81.
13. Lankachandra M, Wells CR, Cheng CJ, et al. Complications of distal phalanx fractures in children. J Hand Surg Am 2017;42(7):574.e1–574.e6.

Mycobacterial Infections in the Hand and Wrist

Abdo Bachoura, MD, David S. Zelouf, MD*

KEYWORDS

- Mycobacteria • Hand infection • Marinum • Tuberculosis • Leprosy

KEY POINTS

- Mycobacterial hand infections usually have an indolent course, marked by variable and nonspecific presentations, often leading to diagnostic and treatment delays.
- The pathogens involved in mycobacterial hand infections include *Mycobacterium tuberculosis* complex, atypical mycobacteria, and *M leprae*.
- Initial treatment involves a combination of long-term antibiotics and surgical débridement to cure the infection.
- Reconstructive procedures aid in restoring hand function lost secondary to the disease process.

BACKGROUND

A majority of hand infections are caused by a few, yet common, gram-positive cocci and gram-negative bacilli. These infections are characterized by significant inflammation and pain, abscess formation, and systemic manifestations. Atypical hand infections are caused by uncommon microbial pathogens, usually have an indolent course, and are marked by variable and nonspecific presentations, often leading to diagnostic and treatment delays. The pathogens responsible for atypical hand infections may be bacterial, fungal, or viral.[1,2] Mycobacterial infections are responsible for a substantial proportion of atypical hand and wrist infections and are the focus of this article.

Mycobacterium is a genus of gram-positive bacilli. These bacteria are nonmotile obligate aerobes that do not form spores. One of the unique features of mycobacteria is their cell wall, which consists of lipoarabinomannan and long-chain fatty acids, called mycolic acids. These molecules give the mycobacteria a hydrophobic cell wall with an unusually high lipid content (greater than 60% of the total cell wall mass).[3] The consistency of the cell wall accounts for many of mycobacteria's biological characteristics and has diagnostic and therapeutic implications. For example, because of the high lipid content, mycobacteria do not stain well with the regular Gram stain method, and the Ziehl-Neelsen technique of acid-fast staining is used for identification.[4] The acid-fast bacillus (AFB) stain is not pathognomonic for mycobacteria, however, because bacteria of the genera *Nocardia*, *Rhodococcus*, *Gordonia*, and *Tsukamurella* also express acid-fast staining characteristics.[4] Mycobacterial treatment is characterized by prolonged antibiotic courses and this is in part related to the hydrophobic cell wall, which makes antibiotic penetration into the cell difficult. Often, a hydrophobic antibiotic (such as rifampin) is included in the antibiotic regimen.[3]

To date, approximately 200 species of mycobacteria have been identified,[5] most of which exist in environmental reservoirs, such as water and soil.[3,4] Conventional phenotypic methods for identification of mycobacteria include observation of colony morphology, pigmentation, biochemical profiles, and rate of growth.[3,4,6] With the ever-increasing number of species identified, however,

The Philadelphia Hand to Shoulder Center, Thomas Jefferson University Hospital, 834 Chestnut Street, Suite G114, Philadelphia, PA 19107, USA
* Corresponding author.
E-mail address: dszelouf@HANDCENTERS.com

Hand Clin 36 (2020) 387–396
https://doi.org/10.1016/j.hcl.2020.03.013

these conventional methods have become less popular among clinical laboratories, because they are laborious and time-consuming, often requiring 6 weeks to 8 weeks for species identification.[4] Newer molecular tests, including polymerase chain reaction (PCR), have become increasingly popular because they are more sensitive and specific than conventional methods and have significantly improved turnaround time.[3,4,7–10]

MYCOBACTERIUM TUBERCULOSIS COMPLEX

Tuberculosis (TB) is a systemic infection caused by a group of similar organisms, referred to as the Mycobacterium tuberculosis complex. The species that make up this complex include M tuberculosis, M africanum, and M bovis.[11] TB was responsible for an estimated 1.3 million deaths among HIV-negative people in 2017 and is the leading cause of death from a single infectious agent.[12] The most common form of TB is a chronic pneumonia with hemoptysis, fever, and weight loss. Musculoskeletal TB usually develops from hematogenous spread of reactivated pulmonary TB or direct inoculation.[13,14] When the hand is affected, however, it frequently is the only site of disease manifestation, and there appears to be an absence of active pulmonary disease in a majority of cases.[15–17]

TB disease presentation in the hand is variable because the infection may involve various soft tissue structures, bones, or joints and may be influenced by the host's cell-mediated immune status. Patients may present with painful or painless volar or dorsal wrist swelling, digital swelling, a discharging wound,[16,17] or axillary or epitrochlear lymphadenopathy.[15,18] Al-Qattan and colleagues[19,20] have classified TB of the hand into the following 6 categories:

1. Cutaneous disease: characterized by nodules that may ulcerate and the subsequent development of lymphadenopathy
2. Tenosynovitis: the most common disease presentation, with the flexors more commonly involved than the extensors[19]
3. Bursitis
4. TB arthritis
5. Osteomyelitis
6. TB hypersensitivity in patients with pulmonary TB, with hand involvement that leads to conditions, such as aseptic arthritis

When suspecting an atypical infection, such as TB, it is important to inquire about a history of exposure, a history of treated TB, or an abnormal chest radiograph.[17] A history of a bloody cough,

unexpected weight loss, or lethargy should raise suspicion. A patient's immune status should be surveyed because immunocompromised patients are more susceptible to reactivation of latent TB.

TB tenosynovitis and arthritis, in particular, are great mimickers and present a diagnostic challenge because they may be confused with more common hand ailments, such as rheumatoid arthritis (RA),[17] carpal tunnel syndrome,[15,17] dorsal ganglion cyst,[17] or de Quervain tenovaginitis.[21] Due to the nonspecific presentation and indolent course of TB in the hand, there are frequent delays between symptom onset, correct diagnosis, and treatment.[17,19] A well-described pitfall accompanying an incorrect diagnosis is corticosteroid injections into the finger or carpal tunnel. This, unfortunately, may exacerbate the infection and lead to worse outcomes.[17]

The diagnostic work-up for a patient with suspected atypical infection of the hand includes blood studies, imaging studies, and eventually incisional or excisional tissue biopsy. When there are no systemic or pulmonary disease manifestations, basic blood studies usually reveal a normal white blood cell count.[16] The erythrocyte sedimentation rate usually is elevated,[17,19] but this not always is the case.[16] Because the initial presentation may be confusing, it is not unreasonable to obtain further blood studies, such as a blood uric acid, rheumatoid factor, antinuclear antibodies, and a Lyme titer.

The TB skin test may have some diagnostic utility as a screening test, because it is inexpensive, has a low morbidity, and has a turnaround time of 48 hours to 72 hours. This test may be falsely negative, however, and it is unclear how sensitive or specific it is for TB of the hand. In their series of 11 patients, Bush and Schneider[17] reported that the TB skin test was negative in 2 out of 2 patients tested, whereas Al-Qattan and colleagues[19] noted falsely negative TB skin tests in several debilitated patients with hand TB. A positive test may indicate that an individual has developed a delayed-type hypersensitivity reaction through infection with mycobacteria (TB or non-TB) at some point in life but does not provide information on whether or not the disease is active. In addition, a positive test may occur in a person who has been immunized with the bacillus Calmette-Guérin vaccine outside of the United States.

TB of the hand most often presents as flexor tenosynovitis and, in this scenario, plain films may reveal nonspecific soft tissue swelling. Late TB osteomyelitis affecting the carpal bones, metacarpals, or phalanges may be unifocal or multifocal and has a variable radiographic appearance, ranging from cystic lesions reminiscent of bone tumors to sclerotic and sometimes sequestrated lesions.[17,19,20] If there are systemic manifestations, such as fatigue, weight loss, or a chronic cough, a chest radiograph may be ordered. In this case, it is appropriate to involve a primary care physician or internal medicine in the overall care of the patient.

If atypical infection is suspected, magnetic resonance imaging (MRI) is recommended because it is capable of providing images of high anatomic definition and readily demonstrates osseous and soft tissue inflammation, synovial thickening, swelling, rice bodies, and fluid collections.[22–24] TB flexor tenosynovitis has no pathognomonic features, and the MRI differential includes giant cell tumor of the tendon sheath.[25] Rice bodies within the flexor tendon sheath may be identified in TB as well as atypical mycobacterial infections and commonly are seen in RA, systemic lupus erythematosus, and seronegative arthritides.[15,17,25,26] Ultrasound also may be useful and has the added benefit of Doppler examination, which may reveal increased vascularity of the involved tendon sheath.[22,23]

The nonspecific clinical presentation and imaging findings may be confusing, especially in countries where TB is uncommon. Under these circumstances, it is reasonable to proceed with an incisional biopsy in order obtain more histologic and microbiological information.[27] Specimens should be sent to the laboratory for histopathologic assessment as well as aerobic, anaerobic, fungal, and mycobacterial culture and stain.[28] Histopathologic findings typically reveal caseating granuloma and Langhans giant cells.[17]

Stains for AFB are negative in most cases of mycobacterial infection.[18,29–31] Prakash and Mehtani[18] reported positive AFB stains in only 19 of 44 pediatric patients (43%) with TB of the hand. TB culture media, such as Middlebrook 7H10 and 7H11 or Löwenstein-Jensen, usually is used, but cultures may take up to 6 weeks to 8 weeks to grow mycobacteria and may not grow any organism.[32] Culture yields as low as 11% have been reported.[18] Although PCR confirmation has been used in equivocal cases,[9,10] a presumptive diagnosis of TB usually is made based on intraoperative and histopathologic findings, despite negative cultures, because this allows initiation of medical treatment.

Treatment of TB in the hand consists of nonsurgical, surgical, or combined treatment. Successful nonoperative treatment of TB flexor tenosynovitis after open incisional biopsy has been reported in a series of 12 patients who underwent 9 months of antibiotic treatment.[15] In this series, the investigators also reported that carpal tunnel symptoms

secondary to TB flexor tenosynovitis resolved after 5 months of treatment.[15] Kotwal and Khan[10] found that nonoperative care was sufficient to treat 24 of 32 (75%) osseous and soft tissue TB hand infections. Patients who did not respond to antibiotic treatment within 8 weeks subsequently underwent surgical débridement. Most investigators, however, report a combination of surgical débridement and antibiotics to cure the infection and to reduce the incidence of recurrence.[9,17,19] Furthermore, early surgery may avoid flexor tendon rupture, although this is a rare and late complication.[9] Surgical indications include a lack of adequate response to medications, hand and wrist deformity, the presence of multiple lesions, and skin ulcerations or sinuses.[15,18] Bush and Schneider[17] reported that inadequate surgical débridement of the diseased tissue, including tenosynovium and bone, may lead to treatment failure. Surgical findings of TB tenosynovitis include the presence of a thick and adherent synovium, which is different from the tenosynovitis seen in RA. Intraoperative surgical findings are helpful in guiding decision making for starting empiric TB antibiotics.[17]

In addition to complete excisional débridement, reconstructive hand surgery plays a role in the treatment of hand TB. For example, 2-stage flexor tendon reconstruction has been performed successfully after débridement of a necrotic flexor tendon,[32] and débridement and arthrodesis of carpal osteomyelitis have been performed successfully.[9]

With regard to antibiotic management, no consensus has been reached about the optimal combination of drugs and duration of treatment. Most treatment regimens range from 6 months to 18 months.[9,18] Because of the high bacterial load and long duration of chemotherapy, the emergence of resistance to isoniazid and rifampin has become a major concern. For this reason, the use of multiple drugs, each with different modes of action, is the standard treatment.[3] The first-line antimycobacterial drugs include isoniazid, ethambutol, rifampin, and pyrazinamide. The second-line drugs are less effective or more toxic than the first-line drugs and include para-aminosalicylic acid, ethionamide, cycloserine, and fluoroquinolones.[3] Second-line drugs may be used in cases of drug resistance. The antibiotic regimen should be managed by an infectious disease specialist for disease control and because long-term antimycobacterial antibiotics may predispose patients to side effects that require frequent monitoring, including hepatotoxicity if isoniazid is used[17] or optic neuritis if ethambutol is used. New cases usually are started on multiple first-line drugs (often all 4) while waiting for results of drug sensitivities. As the results become available, the regimen is adjusted to 2 or 3 active antibiotics.[3]

ATYPICAL MYCOBACTERIA

Atypical mycobacteria also have been referred to as non-TB mycobacteria and as mycobacteria other than tubercle bacilli. These have different colonial characteristics relative to M tuberculosis and are transmitted directly from their environmental reservoirs, such as water and soil.[4,33] Unlike TB, there are no reports of human-to-human transmission. Occurrence in the hand is thought to be related to both the relative abundance of synovium in the region and the increased risk for pathogen inoculation through minor penetrating injuries.[34]

Numerous atypical mycobacterial species may infect the hand and include M marinum, M chelonae, M kansasii, M avium intracellulare complex, M terrae complex, and many others.[24,29,35–42] Up to 93% of patients with atypical mycobacterial hand infections are immunocompetent,[38,43–45] and patients usually do not experience any systemic symptoms. Patients tend to have normal or slightly elevated inflammatory serum markers, such as C-reactive protein.[38] The TB skin test's utility is uncertain for atypical mycobacteria, because it has shown mixed results,[28,46] but may be considered a screening tool.

The nonspecific clinical presentation and imaging findings of atypical mycobacterial hand infections are similar to TB and frequently lead to misdiagnosis and incorrect treatment.[31,37,38] Balagué and colleagues[38] reported a 5.6-month delay in the diagnosis of these infections in the hand. Atypical mycobacterial infections have been mistakenly treated for rheumatological conditions with immunomodulators,[27] carpal tunnel syndrome, cellulitis, abscesses, and arthritis.[28,38,43,44] Unfortunately, inappropriate intralesional steroid injections or oral corticosteroids often lead to worse functional outcomes and may potentiate the infection,[31] resulting in more extensive débridement or amputation and generally worse outcomes (Fig. 1).[29,37,47] A review of 241 cases of non-TB mycobacterial infections, consisting of predominantly M marinum infections (82%), noted that 23% of had received steroid injections prior to the definitive diagnosis.[38]

Similar to cases of TB, atypical mycobacterial AFB stains tend to be negative in a majority of cases.[29–31] Kozin and Bishop[30] found that only 30% of atypical mycobacteria infections stained positive. The classic histologic finding is a noncaseating granuloma on hematoxylin-eosin

stain[24,47,48] or on a frozen section.[24] Granulomatous disease identified on microscopy, however, is a nonspecific finding and may be misleading if not correlated with the clinical presentation and culture results (see Fig. 1). Owing to the fastidious nature of mycobacteria and the prolonged incubation time, culture yields for atypical mycobacteria may be as low as 42%.[31,49] When the cultures are negative, a presumptive diagnosis may be made based on a history of exposure, occupational risk, clinical examination, surgical findings (rice bodies), and histopathologic findings of granulomatous inflammation.[31,38,46] Although PCR has been used for atypical mycobacteria detection,[23,49] clinical laboratories may have different testing protocols and may not have this advanced test available. Therefore, when clinical suspicion for atypical bacterial infection is high, it may be beneficial for the surgeon to communicate directly with the laboratory to determine the testing requirements and capacities of the laboratory.

Surgically treated patients who are not treated with concomitant antibiotics have a poor functional prognosis,[38] and appropriate antibiotics should be started as soon as the operative findings are consistent with atypical infection.[44] There still is no standard antimicrobial therapy for atypical mycobacterial infection. Clinical isolates should be sent for sensitivity testing due to variable drug susceptibility. Atypical antimycobacterial treatment varies and usually is given for 5 months to 12 months,[27,31,38] although some studies have reported a 1-month course.[43] Patients should be advised that clinical success is not expected to be immediate. The first signs of substantial improvement may be observed at a median of 3 months.[38]

Mycobacterium marinum

M marinum infection predominantly infects the hand and upper extremity.[38,50] Among the atypical mycobacteria infecting the hand, M marinum is the most common pathogen, accounting for 41% to 82% of cases.[38,43,50] The optimal temperature for M marinum growth is 30°C to 3°C and this may explain the infection's predilection for the hands, which generally are cooler than the core body temperature. Disease transmission of M marinum occurs when the patient sustains a puncture wound or abrasion by contaminated fish, shrimp, oysters, or other aquatic animals or has an open wound exposed to contaminated water (Fig. 2). Both fresh water and salt water may harbor M marinum, and most reports describe a history of fish handling or household aquarium cleaning.[50]

The clinical manifestations typically are localized to the hand and vary substantially because

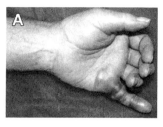
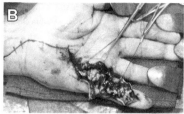

Fig. 1. (*A*) 68-year-old man who initially presented with carpal tunnel syndrome symptoms. He underwent open carpal tunnel release, where the tenosynovial tissue was noted to be abnormal. The tenosynovium was biopsied but not cultured. Permanent section showed inflammatory disease, most consistent with RA. The patient was prescribed prednisone, 40 mg daily, for 3 months. Patient was seen by rheumatology at 3 months with swollen and extended small finger as well as mild pain and swelling at the A1 pulley of the thumb. (*B*) The patient was brought to the operating room that night. Extensive flexor tenosynovitis was observed. He underwent radical débridement, including débridement of Parona space and a horseshoe abscess that tracked into the thumb. The patient underwent multiple débridements and finally a small finger amputation. *M marinum* was confirmed on culture. Upon further questioning, the patient confirmed sustaining a fish hook injury to the small fingertip many months before his presentation.

both superficial and deep structures may be involved to various extents. Skin involvement may appear as single or multiple nodular, papulo-verrucous, pustular, ulcerative lesions or as a draining sinus.[35–37] Spread may occur along the lymphatics, resulting in a sporotrichoid pattern, reminiscent of a sporotrichosis fungal infection.[50]

Therefore, examination of the epitrochlear and axillary lymph nodes is important to fully appreciate the disease presentation. Deep infection with *M marinum* may lead to bursitis, synovitis, flexor tenosynovitis and rice body formation,[23] extensor tenosynovitis,[37] septic arthritis, or osteomyelitis.[51]

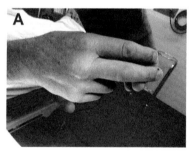
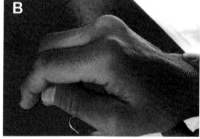
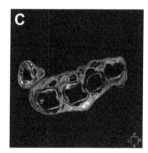
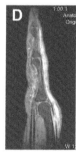
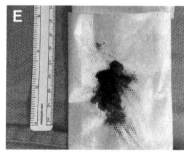

Fig. 2. (*A*, *B*) A 62-year old man presented in January 2019, with a 1-month history of spontaneous onset swelling and pain of his right middle finger. He did not have any systemic symptoms, and he had not responded to colchicine or amoxicillin. (*C*, *D*) Axial and sagittal T2-weighted MRIs revealed a small multiloculated fluid collection with central debris within the dorsal subcutaneous tissue at the level of the metacarpal head, with mild reactive extensor tenosynovitis and subcutaneous edema concerning for infection. (*E*) Intraoperatively, exuberant tenosynovitis, superficial to the extensor tendon, was observed. Histopathology revealed granulomatous inflammation. The patient recalled sustaining multiple hand abrasions while standing in a river and removing barnacles from a boat 4 months prior to the onset of his symptoms. The patient was referred to infectious disease and given a putative diagnosis of *M marinum* infection based on his history, intraoperative findings, and histopathology. AFB stain was negative and cultures did not grow any organisms. He was treated with 3 months of clarithromycin, rifampin, and ethambutol and made a full recovery.

Superficial or cutaneous marinum infection may be treated effectively with antibiotics; however, deep infection is more resistant to nonoperative treatment.[37] The aims of surgery generally are to obtain adequate tissue for biopsy and cultures and to remove as much disease as possible. Failure of *M marinum* treatment has been related to deep involvement.[50] It is thought that excisional débridement debulks the infected and necrotic tissue and allows for better antimicrobial penetration. Although uncommon, fluid collections, purulence, and a discharging sinus may be present in marinum infection and have been treated effectively by surgical decompression in addition to antibiotics.[37,45] Amputation or ray resection may be performed for nonfunctional, painful, and stiff digits or for disease control.[38,52] After surgery, antibiotic treatment and follow-up with an infectious disease specialist are recommended and patients should be monitored closely because it is not uncommon to require multiple débridements.[31,52]

Mycobacterium chelonae

The natural reservoirs of *M chelonae* include soil, water, animals, and marine life.[4] *M chelonae* is classified as a rapidly growing non-TB mycobacteria (grows within 7 days)[3,4,29] and may infect both immunocompromised[40] and, more commonly, immunocompetent patients.[29,53] In immunocompetent patients, clinical presentation is similar to that with other atypical mycobacteria and usually is flexor tenosynovitis, with no systemic symptoms and normal basic blood work. *M chelonae* may be resistant to doxycycline and rifampin and susceptible to clarithromycin.[29,53] Combined surgical and medical treatment usually is necessary, and, although most patients recover completely, amputation and ray resection have been reported for disease control.[29,39]

Mycobacterium kansasii

The natural reservoirs of *M kansasii* include water and cattle.[4] *M kansasii* usually presents as a lung infection, similar to TB presentation,[54] but may infect both immunocompetent and immunocompromised hosts. In the hand, *M kansasii* often manifests as flexor tenosynovitis, but osteomyelitis of the scaphoid also has been reported.[55,56] Combined surgical and medical treatment usually is recommended. Resistance to rifampin and ethambutol has been reported.[56]

Mycobacterium avium Complex

M avium complex (MAC) is a common cause of systemic bacterial infection in patients with the acquired immunodeficiency syndrome.[4,57] The natural reservoirs include soil, water, birds, fowl, swine, and cattle. MAC refers to organisms identified as *M avium* and *M intracellulare*. In immunocompetent patients, MAC has been identified as a cause of pulmonary infection in adults. It also may cause soft tissue infections in the hands of immunocompetent individuals and is treated similarly, with a combination of surgery and medications.[58]

MAC tends to exhibit resistance to isoniazid and pyrazinamide. There are few clinical data to guide therapy, but a combination of clarithromycin or azithromycin, ethambutol, and rifampin or rifabutin is used in the treatment of pulmonary MAC disease and presumably should be used in the treatment of tenosynovitis.[24]

MYCOBACTERIUM LEPRAE

Leprosy, also known as Hansen disease, is a chronic granulomatous disease of the skin and peripheral nerves. It is caused by *M leprae* and, if left untreated, can cause progressive and permanent damage to the skin, peripheral nerves, limbs, and eyes.[59] Fortunately, 95% of the human population is not susceptible to infection with *M leprae* and treatment with multidrug therapy in the early stages can prevent disability and lead to a cure.[59,60] Leprosy remains endemic in certain parts of Asia, South America, and Africa. In nonendemic areas, where health care providers do not have sufficient experience with this disease, the clinical picture may be confused with rheumatological conditions or fungal infections and often leads to delayed treatment.[61,62] The disease is thought to occur primarily through human-to-human droplet transmission, but zoonotic disease spread via armadillos also is possible.[3,4,61,63]

Diagnosis of leprosy is primarily clinical and is confirmed by demonstration of AFB in Fite-stained scrapings of infected tissue.[3,4] Biopsy of skin or of a thickened nerve revealing AFB also may be helpful in establishing the diagnosis.[4,64] Efforts to grow the organism in the laboratory setting have remained unsuccessful to date.[4]

Patient immunity is responsible for the presenting form of leprosy. There are 2 major forms, tuberculoid and lepromatous, with a spectrum of illness in between.[65] Tuberculoid leprosy is indolent and is paucibacilliary. This form of the disease usually is noncontagious and characterized by the development of macules or plaques on the face, trunk, and limbs and dry, pale, hairless centers. When peripheral nerves are invaded, the lesions become insensate.[3,65] In lepromatous leprosy, skin lesions are infiltrative and extensive, and peripheral

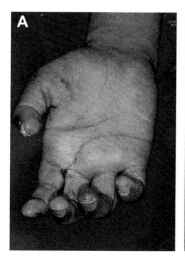
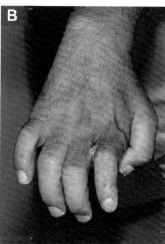

Fig. 3. (*A, B*) A 22-year-old man from Micronesia with severe median and ulnar neuropathy secondary to recently diagnosed *M leprae*. (*Courtesy of* B. F. Plucknette, DO, DPT, Maj, USAF, MC, San Antonio, TX.)

neuropathies may produce deformities or non-healing painless ulcers (**Fig. 3**).[3,65] *M leprae* targets both myelinating and nonmyelinating forms of Schwann cells, and, if left untreated, the infection leads to demyelination, nerve fiber degeneration, and fibrosis.[3,64–66] The ulnar nerve is by far the most commonly affected peripheral nerve in the upper extremity,[67] followed by the median nerve and least commonly the radial nerve.[68,69] Loss of the sensations of pain and temperature predisposes patients to frequent injury, which subsequently leads to osteomyelitis, gangrene, and loss of digits.[67]

Multidrug therapy with dapsone is the first-line of treatment of both tuberculoid leprosy and lepromatous leprosy.[3] Rifampin and clofazimine generally are included in the antibiotic regimen. Additional medications used include minocycline, clarithromycin, and certain fluoroquinolones. In order to treat leprosy adequately, medications may have to be used for several months to years.[3] Patients may develop immunologically mediated inflammation in response to the dead bacilli antigens before, during, or after multidrug therapy.[70,71] These leprosy reactions can present as neuritis, fevers, arthralgias, or painful skin lesions and are capable of causing additional peripheral nerve damage and disability.[62] Treatment of leprosy reactions usually is with oral corticosteroids.[62,71]

Surgical treatment of leprosy in the upper extremity includes nerve decompression,[72–75] abscess evacuation, contracture releases, and reconstructive surgery.[68] Restoration of sensibility and autonomic function with the use of digital nerve transfers has been performed with favorable outcomes,[76] but a majority of elective reconstructive hand surgery are performed to treat motor paralysis with the use of tendon transfers.[67,68,77,78]

SUMMARY

Mycobacterial infections in the hand and wrist remain a diagnostic and therapeutic challenge because of their low incidence and ability to mimic more common hand conditions. Although management of these infections is based on a team approach, which involves both medical and surgical treatments, the hand surgeon may be one of the first health care providers to encounter these infections. Therefore, a high index of suspicion for mycobacterial hand infections should be maintained, in particular with an unusual patient presentation or a puzzling constellation of signs and symptoms.

DISCLOSURE

The authors have nothing to disclose.

REFERENCES

1. Hoyen HA, Lacey SH, Graham TJ. Atypical hand infections. Hand Clin 1998;14:613–34.
2. Chan E, Bagg M. Atypical Hand Infections. Orthop Clin North Am 2017;48:229–40.
3. Mycobacteria. In: Ryan KJ, editors. Sherris medical microbiology, 7th edition. New York: McGraw-Hill. Available at: http://accessmedicine.mhmedical.com/content.aspx?bookid=2268&sectionid=176086056. Accessed June 30, 2019.
4. Mycobacteria. In: Riedel S, Hobden JA, Miller S, et al, editors. Jawetz, Melnick, & Adelberg's medical microbiology, 28th edition. New York: McGraw-Hill.

Available at: http://accessmedicine.mhmedical.com/content.aspx?bookid=2629&sectionid=217771812. Accessed June 30, 2019.

5. Available at: http://www.bacterio.net/mycobacterium.html. Accessed June 30, 2019.

6. Runyon EH. Pathogenic mycobacteria. Adv Tuberc Res 1965;14:235.

7. Somoskovi A, Mester J, Hale YM, et al. Laboratory diagnosis of nontuberculous mycobacteria. Clin Chest Med 2002;23:585–97.

8. Abdalla CM, de Oliveira ZN, Sotto MN, et al. Polymerase chain reaction compared to other laboratory findings and to clinical evaluation in the diagnosis of cutaneous tuberculosis and atypical mycobacteria skin infection. Int J Dermatol 2009;48:27–35.

9. Woon CY, Phoon ES, Lee JY, et al. Rice bodies, millet seeds, and melon seeds in tuberculous tenosynovitis of the hand and wrist. Ann Plast Surg 2011;66:610–7.

10. Kotwal PP, Khan SA. Tuberculosis of the hand: clinical presentation and functional outcome in 32 patients. J Bone Joint Surg Br 2009;91:1054–7.

11. Sharma A, Bloss E, Heilig CM, et al. Tuberculosis Caused by Mycobacterium africanum, United States, 2004-2013. Emerg Infect Dis 2016;22:396–403.

12. Global tuberculosis report 2018. Geneva (Switzerland): World Health Organization; 2018. Licence: CC BY-NC-SA 3.0 IGO.

13. Pattamapaspong N, Muttarak M, Sivasomboon C. Tuberculosis arthritis and tenosynovitis. Semin Musculoskelet Radiol 2011;15:459–69.

14. Celikyay F, Yuksekkaya RZ, Bostan B. Flexor tenosynovitis of the wrist including rice bodies. Joint Bone Spine 2018;85:373.

15. Kabakaş F, Uğurlar M, Turan DB, et al. Flexor Tenosynovitis Due to Tuberculosis in Hand and Wrist: Is Tenosynovectomy Imperative? Ann Plast Surg 2016;77:169–72.

16. Ritz N, Connell TG, Tebruegge M, et al. Tuberculous dactylitis–an easily missed diagnosis. Eur J Clin Microbiol Infect Dis 2011;30:1303–10.

17. Bush DC, Schneider LH. Tuberculosis of the hand and wrist. J Hand Surg Am 1984;9:391–8.

18. Prakash J, Mehtani A. Hand and wrist tuberculosis in paediatric patients - our experience in 44 patients. J Pediatr Orthop B 2017;26:250–60.

19. Al-Qattan MM, Al-Namla A, Al-Thunayan A, et al. Tuberculosis of the hand. J Hand Surg Am 2011;36:1413–21.

20. Al-Qattan MM, Helmi AA. Chronic hand infections. J Hand Surg Am 2014;39:1636–45.

21. Chen WS, Eng HL. Tuberculous tenosynovitis of the wrist mimicking de Quervain's disease. J Rheumatol 1994;21:763–5.

22. Soldatos T, Omar H, Sammer D, et al. Atypical Infections versus Inflammatory Conditions of the Hand: The Role of Imaging in Diagnosis. Plast Reconstr Surg 2015;136:316–27.

23. Sanal HT, Zor F, Kocaoğlu M, et al. Atypical mycobacterial tenosynovitis and bursitis of the wrist. Diagn Interv Radiol 2009;15:266–8.

24. Anim-Appiah D, Bono B, Fleegler E, et al. Mycobacterium avium complex tenosynovitis of the wrist and hand. Arthritis Rheum 2004;51:140–2.

25. Tyllianakis M, Kasimatis G, Athanaselis S, et al. Rice-body formation and tenosynovitis of the wrist: a case report. J Orthop Surg (Hong Kong) 2006;14:208–11.

26. Cheung HS, Ryan LM, Kozin F, et al. Synovial origins of Rice bodies in joint fluid. Arthritis Rheum 1980;23:72–6.

27. Beam E, Vasoo S, Simner PJ, et al. Mycobacterium arupense flexor tenosynovitis: case report and review of antimicrobial susceptibility profiles for 40 clinical isolates. J Clin Microbiol 2014;52:2706–8.

28. Gunther SF, Elliott RC, Brand RL, et al. Experience with atypical mycobacterial infection in the deep structures of the hand. J Hand Surg Am 1977;2:90–6.

29. Lee EY, Ip JW, Fung BK, et al. Mycobacterium chelonae hand infection: a review. Hand Surg 2009;14:7–13.

30. Kozin SH, Bishop AT. Atypical Mycobacterium infections of the upper extremity. J Hand Surg Am 1994;19:480–7.

31. Cheung JP, Fung BK, Ip WY. Mycobacterium marinum infection of the deep structures of the hand and wrist: 25 years of experience. Hand Surg 2010;15:211–6.

32. Karunadasa KP, Dissanayake DA, Beneragama TS, et al. Staged flexor tendon reconstruction in a patient with caseous tuberculous tenosynovitis. J Hand Surg Eur Vol 2010;35:515–6.

33. Katoch VM. Infections due to non-tuberculous mycobacteria (NTM). Indian J Med Res 2004;120:290–304.

34. Theodorou DJ, Theodorou SJ, Kakitsubata Y, et al. Imaging characteristics and epidemiologic features of atypical mycobacterial infections involving the musculoskeletal system. AJR Am J Roentgenol 2001;176:341–9.

35. Bonamonte D, De Vito D, Vestita M, et al. Aquarium-borne Mycobacterium marinum skin infection. Report of 15 cases and review of the literature. Eur J Dermatol 2013;23:510–6.

36. Huminer D, Pitlik SD, Block C, et al. Aquarium-borne Mycobacterium marinum skin infection. Report of a case and review of the literature. Arch Dermatol 1986;122:698–703.

37. Chow SP, Ip FK, Lau JH, et al. Mycobacterium marinum infection of the hand and wrist. Results of conservative treatment in twenty-four cases. J Bone Joint Surg Am 1987;69:1161–8.

38. Balagué N, Uçkay I, Vostrel P, et al. Non-tuberculous mycobacterial infections of the hand. Chir Main 2015;34:18–23.

39. Stern PJ, Gula DC. Mycobacterium chelonei tenosynovitis of the hand: a case report. J Hand Surg Am 1986;11:596–9.

40. Iyengar KP, Nadkarni JB, Gupta R, et al. Mycobacterium chelonae hand infection following ferret bite. Infection 2013;41:237–41.

41. Gunther SF, Elliott RC. Mycobacterium kansasii infection in the deep structures of the hand. Report of two cases. J Bone Joint Surg Am 1976;58:140–2.

42. Namkoong H, Fukumoto K, Hongo I, et al. Refractory tenosynovitis with 'rice bodies' in the hand due to Mycobacterium intracellulare. Infection 2016;44: 393–4.

43. Lopez M, Croley J, Murphy KD. Atypical mycobacterial infections of the upper extremity: becoming more atypical? Hand (N Y) 2017;12:188–92.

44. Brutus JP, Baeten Y, Chahidi N, et al. Atypical mycobacterial infections of the hand: report of eight cases and literature review. Chir Main 2001;20:280–6.

45. Pang HN, Lee JY, Puhaindran ME, et al. Mycobacterium marinum as a cause of chronic granulomatous tenosynovitis in the hand. J Infect 2007;54: 584–8.

46. Lewis FM, Marsh BJ, von Reyn CF. Fish tank exposure and cutaneous infections due to Mycobacterium marinum: tuberculin skin testing, treatment, and prevention. Clin Infect Dis 2003;37:390–7.

47. Wada A, Nomura S, Ihara F. Mycobacterium kansaii flexor tenosynovitis presenting as carpal tunnel syndrome. J Hand Surg Br 2000;25:308–10.

48. Hurst LC, Amadio PC, Badalamente MA, et al. Mycobacterium marinum infections of the hand. J Hand Surg Am 1987;12:428–35.

49. Ehrlichman LK, Kadzielski JJ, Hyle EP, et al. Nontuberculous Mycobacterial Osteomyelitis of the Thumb: Successful Treatment with Serial Debridement, Antimicrobial Therapy, External Fixation, and Interphalangeal Arthrodesis: A Case Report. JBJS Case Connect 2015;5:e87.

50. Aubry A, Chosidow O, Caumes E, et al. Sixty-three cases of Mycobacterium marinum infection: clinical features, treatment, and antibiotic susceptibility of causative isolates. Arch Intern Med 2002;162: 1746–52.

51. Clark RB, Spector H, Friedman DM, et al. Osteomyelitis and synovitis produced by Mycobacterium marinum in a fisherman. J Clin Microbiol 1990;28: 2570–2.

52. Wendt JR, Lamm RC, Altman DI, et al. An unusually aggressive Mycobacterium marinum hand infection. J Hand Surg Am 1986;11:753–5.

53. Mateo L, Rufí G, Nolla JM, et al. Mycobacterium chelonae tenosynovitis of the hand. Semin Arthritis Rheum 2004;34:617–22.

54. DeStefano MS, Shoen CM, Cynamon MH. Therapy for mycobacterium kansasii infection: beyond 2018. Front Microbiol 2018;9:2271.

55. Wang MS, Berry M, Lehto-Hoffman A, et al. Chronic Tenosynovitis due to Mycobacteria kansasii in an Immunocompetent Host. Case Rep Infect Dis 2018;2018:3297531.

56. Minkin BI, Mills CL, Bullock DW, et al. Mycobacterium kansasii osteomyelitis of the scaphoid. J Hand Surg Am 1987;12:1092–4.

57. Lugo-Janer G, Cruz A, Sánchez JL. Disseminated cutaneous infection caused by Mycobacterium avium complex. Arch Dermatol 1990;126:1108–10.

58. Hellinger WC, Smilack JD, Greider JL Jr, et al. Localized soft-tissue infections with Mycobacterium avium/Mycobacterium intracellulare complex in immunocompetent patients: granulomatous tenosynovitis of the hand or wrist. Clin Infect Dis 1995; 21:65–9.

59. World Health Organization. Available at: https://www.who.int/news-room/fact-sheets/detail/leprosy. Accessed July 4, 2019.

60. Health Resources and Services Administration. Available at: https://www.hrsa.gov/hansens-disease/index.html. Accessed July 6, 2019.

61. Aslam S, Peraza J, Mekaiel A, et al. Major risk factors for leprosy in a non-endemic area of the United States: a case series. IDCases 2019;17:e00557.

62. Leon KE, Salinas JL, McDonald RW. Complex type 2 reactions in three patients with Hansen's disease from a Southern United States Clinic. Am J Trop Med Hyg 2015;93:1082–6.

63. Truman RW, Singh P, Sharma R, et al. Probable zoonotic leprosy in the southern United States. N Engl J Med 2011;364:1626–33.

64. Payne R, Baccon J, Dossett J, et al. Pure neuritic leprosy presenting as ulnar nerve neuropathy: a case report of electrodiagnostic, radiographic, and histopathological findings. J Neurosurg 2015;123: 1238–43.

65. Ridley DS, Jopling WH. Classification of leprosy according to immunity: a five group system. Int J Lepr Other Mycobact Dis 1966;34:255–73.

66. Chan JP, Uong J, Nassiri N, et al. Lessons from leprosy: peripheral neuropathies and deformities in chronic demyelinating diseases. J Hand Surg Am 2019;44:411–5.

67. Brand PW. The reconstruction of the hand in leprosy. Ann R Coll Surg Engl 1952;11:350–61.

68. Anderson GA. The surgical management of deformities of the hand in leprosy. J Bone Joint Surg Br 2006;88:290–4.

69. Sundararaj GD, Mani K. Surgical reconstruction of the hand with triple nerve palsy. J Bone Joint Surg Br 1984;66:260–4.

70. Mowla MR, Ara S, Mizanur Rahman AFM, et al. Leprosy reactions in postelimination stage: the

Bangladesh experience. J Eur Acad Dermatol Venereol 2017;31:705–11.

71. Bernink EH, Voskens JE. Study on the detection of leprosy reactions and the effect of prednisone on various nerves, Indonesia. Lepr Rev 1997;68:225–32.

72. Wan EL, Rivadeneira AF, Jouvin RM, et al. Treatment of Peripheral Neuropathy in Leprosy: The Case for Nerve Decompression. Plast Reconstr Surg Glob Open 2016;4:e637.

73. Pannikar VK, Ramprasad S, Reddy NR, et al. Effect of epicondylectomy in early ulnar neuritis treated with steroids. Int J Lepr Other Mycobact Dis 1984;52:501–5.

74. Ebenezer M, Andrews P, Solomon S. Comparative trial of steroids and surgical intervention in the management of ulnar neuritis. Int J Lepr Other Mycobact Dis 1996;64:282–6.

75. Van Veen NH, Schreuders TA, Theuvenet WJ, et al. Decompressive surgery for treating nerve damage in leprosy. Cochrane Database Syst Rev 2012;(12):CD006983.

76. Ozkan T, Ozer K, Gülgönen A. Restoration of sensibility in irreparable ulnar and median nerve lesions with use of sensory nerve transfer: long-term follow-up of 20 cases. J Hand Surg Am 2001;26:44–51.

77. Rath S. Split flexor pollicis longus tendon transfer to A1 pulley for correction of paralytic Z deformity of the thumb. J Hand Surg Am 2013;38:1172–80.

78. Mohammed AK, Lalonde DH. Wide awake tendon transfers in leprosy patients in India. Hand Clin 2019;35:67–84.

Printed and bound by CPI Group (UK) Ltd, Croydon, CR0 4YY

03/10/2024

01040372-0007